Infectious Diseases and Microbiology

snova
New York

Infectious Diseases and Microbiology

Psychological Consequences of the COVID-19 Pandemic on Children, Teenagers and Adults
Jean-Pascal Assailly, PhD (Editor)
2022. ISBN: 978-1-68507-963-5 (Softcover)
2022. ISBN: 979-8-88697-072-2 (eBook)

COVID-19 Contracting: Opportunities, Actions and Reimbursements
Eric Neudorf
2022. ISBN: 978-1-68507-710-5 (Hardcover)
2022. ISBN: 978-1-68507-733-4 (eBook)

The Aviation Industry and COVID-19
Stefan Schneider
2022. ISBN: 978-1-68507-712-9 (Hardcover)
2022. ISBN: 978-1-68507-729-7 (eBook)

Diseases Transmitted by Ticks
Hacer İşler, Metin Özdemir, MD (Editors)
2021. ISBN: 978-1-68507-359-6 (Hardcover)
2021. ISBN: 978-1-68507-383-1 (eBook)

Impacts and Implications of COVID-19: An Analytical and Empirical Study
Anand Sharma, Prateek Agrawal, Vishu Madaan, Anuj Agarwal (Editors)
2021. ISBN: 978-1-53619-670-2 (Hardcover)
2021. ISBN: 978-1-68507-081-6 (eBook)

More information about this series can be found at https://novapublishers.com/product-category/series/infectious-diseases-and-microbiology/

Richard D. Hylton
Editor

A Closer Look at the COVID-19 Variants

snova
New York

Library of Congress Cataloging-in-Publication Data

ISBN: 979-8-88697-170-5

Published by Nova Science Publishers, Inc. † New York

Contents

Preface

As viruses spread, small errors - called mutations - arise in the genetic material during replication. Many of these mutations are repaired or die off as the virus continues to move through a population. Mutations that enhance the virus's ability to replicate, transmit, or survive in a host allow the virus to spread more quickly through a population, or become more resistant to immune system defenses, thereby increasing the mutations' prevalence and creating a new strain of the virus.

The purpose of this book is to discuss how variants develop, how researchers identify and sequence variants, and how this information can be utilized by public health officials, government agencies, and medical practitioners to make decisions. The book examines the ways the government can better coordinate its approach to best serve the American people through this pandemic and beyond.

Chapter 1

COVID–19 Variants and Evolving Research Needs*

Committee on Science, Space, and Technology

Wednesday, May 12, 2021
House of Representatives,
Subcommittee on Investigations and Oversight,
Committee on Science, Space, and Technology,
Washington, D.C.

The Subcommittee met, pursuant to notice, at 10:03 a.m., via Zoom, Hon. Bill Foster [Chairman of the Subcommittee] presiding.

Purpose

The purpose of this hearing is to discuss how variants develop, how researchers identify and sequence variants, and how this information can be utilized by public health officials, government agencies, and medical practitioners to make decisions. The hearing will examine the ways the Federal government can meet the research and forecasting needs that evolve as the virus continues to mutate. Members and witnesses will discuss how the federal government can better coordinate its approach to best serve the American people through this pandemic and beyond.

* This is an edited, reformatted and augmented version of Hearing before the Subcommittee on Investigations and Oversight of the Committee on Science, Space, and Technology House of Representatives, Serial No. 117–14, dated May 12, 2021.

In: A Closer Look at the COVID-19 Variants
Editor: Richard D. Hylton
ISBN: 979-8-88697-170-5

Witnesses

- Dr. Salim Abdool Karim, Director of CAPRISA
- Dr. Nathan Grubaugh, Assistant Professor of Epidemiology, Yale School of Public Health
- Dr. Stephen Streiffer, Deputy Laboratory Director for Science and Technology, Argonne National Laboratory
- Dr. Caitlin Rivers, Senior Scholar, Johns Hopkins Center for Health Security

Overarching Questions

- How do COVID-19 variants emerge and spread, and how do public health decisionsinfluence the proliferation of variants?
- What is the state of data sharing among U.S. states and among countries regardingvariants developing and spreading around the globe?
- Are existing tests and vaccines effective for the known COVID-19 variants? How do variant-specific tests bolster public health decision-making? What role do vaccines playin reducing the spread and emergence of variants?
- Have the models built to track and predict the spread of COVID-19 around the globeadapted with the emergence and spread of variants?
- How can the federal government serve as a resource during and between pandemics whenit comes to information aggregation and accessibility and disease forecasting?

Variants in the United States

As viruses spread, small errors – called mutations – arise in the genetic material during replication. Many of these mutations are repaired or die off as the virus continues to move through a population. Mutations that enhance the virus's ability to replicate, transmit, or survive in a host allow the virus to spread more quickly through a population, or become more resistant to immune system defenses, thereby increasing the mutations' prevalence and creating a new strain of the virus.[1] Almost a year and a half into the global battle against COVID-19, the United States faces five known Variants of Concern (VOCs). According to the Centers for Disease Control,[2] these are as follows:

- B.1.1.7: First identified in the U.K. in November 2020 and identified in the U.S. in December 2020. This variant increased transmissibility of the virus by about 50% and research suggests there is a potential – but not confirmed – increase in severity of cases.[3]
- B.1.351: First identified in South Africa in December 2020 and identified I the U.S. at the end of January 2021. This variant increased transmissibility of the virus by about 50%. Certain monoclonal antibody treatments and vaccine-induced immunity have been shown to be less effective against B.1.351.[4]
- P.1: First identified in Japan in early January 2021 among travelers from Brazil, where it likely originated in November 2020.[5] Identified in the U.S. in January 2021. Research indicates P.1 is twice as transmissible as earlier strains and is less susceptible to immune defenses built by previous infections and vaccination.[6]
- B.1.427 and B.1.429: First identified in California in February 2021. This variant increased transmissibility of the virus by about 20%. Certain monoclonal antibody treatments and vaccine-induced immunity have been shown to be less effective against these variants.[7]

As variants of concern, these strains have evidence of an increase in transmissibility, more severe disease, significant reduction in susceptibility to infection- or vaccine-induced immunity, or diagnostic detection failures.[8] These variants are closely monitored by federal health agencies and are analyzed to determine whether additional diagnostics, vaccines, or treatment

---

[1] https://www.gavi.org/vaccineswork/patient-zero-understanding-how-new-coronavirus-variants-emerge.

[2] https://www.cdc.gov/coronavirus/2019-ncov/transmission/variant.html.

[3] https://www.cdc.gov/coronavirus/2019-ncov/cases-updates/variant-surveillance/variant-info.html.

[4] Ibid.

[5] https://www.sciencenews.org/article/covid-coronavirus-p1-variant-brazil-strain-transmission-immunity.

[6] Ibis.

[7] https://www.cdc.gov/coronavirus/2019-ncov/cases-updates/variant-surveillance/variant-info.html.

[8] Ibid.

are needed. If clear evidence of reduced effectiveness of prevention measures, vaccines, or approved therapeutics arises, a variant could be classified as a Variant of High Consequence. Currently, no COVID-19 variants rise to this level.

B.1.617 and the Importance of Vaccines in Squelching Variants

The variant currently dominating the news cycle was discovered in India. India is now experiencing the sharpest spike in coronavirus cases in the world, with a record of 400,000 new COVID-19 cases for the first time on May 1.[9] One variant – B.1.617 – has become the dominant strain in some areas. Media coverage of this variant has dubbed it a "double mutant," as it contains specific similarities to the mutation present in the California strain as well as one found in both the South African and Brazilian strains. However, this name implies that the strain has only two mutations, or that having two mutations is unusual; in fact, B.1.617 has about a dozen mutations, which is not uncommon.[10]

While B.1.617 is not the only mutation driving up infections in India, it appears that people who already had COVID-19 during an earlier surge are susceptible to reinfection with B.1.617.

Existing vaccines appear to work against B.1.617, but could be slightly less effective.[11]

Exacerbating this deadly wave in India is the country's vaccine shortage. India is the largest vaccine manufacturer in the world, but just about 3 percent of the country – 30 million out of 1.3 billion people – had been fully vaccinated as of May 8.[12] Expanding vaccine access is not only imperative to save lives in India during this devastating wave, but to stem the spread of the virus and the inevitable mutations that will develop as it makes its way through the population. In late April, the Biden administration announced that it would share 60 million doses of the AstraZeneca vaccine – which is not authorized

---

[9] https://www.reuters.com/world/asia-pacific/india-posts-record-daily-rise-covid-19-cases-401993-2021-05-01/.

[10] https://www.npr.org/sections/goatsandsoda/2021/04/24/988744811/people-are-talking-about-a-double-mutant- variant-in-india-what-does-that-mean.

[11] Ibid.

[12] https://www.nytimes.com/live/2021/05/06/world/covid-vaccine-coronavirus-cases.

for use in the United States by the Food and Drug Administration (FDA) – with countries around the world.[13]

On May 5, 2021, the Administration announced that it supports the temporary lifting of intellectual property protections for COVID-19 vaccines.[14] Lifting these protections would allow the production of generic versions of the vaccines to supplement the doses made available directly from brand-name pharmaceutical companies, from other countries, or through international programs such as COVAX, which aims to provide equitable access to tests, treatments, and vaccines.[15] Pharmaceutical companies are opposed to lifting these protections, arguing that the increased competition for supplies could slow their production.

The more the virus circulates, the more variants will emerge, increasing the risk of a deadlier, more contagious strain of the disease. Though the exact effectiveness varies among vaccines and among variants, all approved vaccines appear to be effective in preventing infection from known variants. Last week, studies were published that showed the Pfizer-BioNTech vaccine to be 100 percent effective at preventing severe disease caused by B.1.351 (South African variant) and B.1.1.7 (U.K. variant), and 72-89.5 percent effective at preventing infection.[16] Suppressing the spread and inevitable mutation of the coronavirus – especially as the world is opening back up – requires robust vaccination in the United States and abroad.[17]

Variant Testing

Though the tests used to detect the coronavirus were developed in the flurry of the early days of the pandemic, there is no evidence that they are less effective at detecting the newer strains of the virus.[18] Polymerase chain reaction tests – or PCR tests – detect multiple sequences of the coronavirus genome. The detection of any one of these sequences will trigger a positive

---

[13] https://www.washingtonpost.com/politics/us-to-share-up-to-60-million-doses-of-astrazeneca-coronavirus-vaccine- with-other-countries-official-says/2021/04/26/b2dab8a0-a694-11eb-bca5-048b2759a489_story.html.

[14] https://twitter.com/ambassadortai/status/1390021205974003720?s=21.

[15] https://www.who.int/initiatives/act-accelerator/covax.

[16] https://www.nytimes.com/live/2021/05/05/world/covid-vaccine-coronavirus-ca ses#pfizer-vaccine-variants-covid.

[17] https://www.seattletimes.com/opinion/rise-of-variants-underscores-importance-of-covid-19-vaccination/.

[18] https://www.nytimes.com/2021/04/14/health/coronavirus-testing-variants.html.

test result, meaning that the mutation of one gene target will not render the test ineffective. However, it is important that researchers, test manufacturers, and regulatory bodies remain vigilant in assessing the continued effectiveness of tests as the virus continues to mutate. The FDA maintains a list of EUA-authorized tests whose performance may be impacted by mutations,[19] and has issued policy guidance and recommendations for evaluating the impact of variants on tests.[20]

Because certain variants are deadlier, more contagious, or respond differently to preventative measures or treatments, it is important that public health agencies understand where particular variants are emerging and circulating. While not in use diagnostically, genomic sequencing is used to identify specific strains of the coronavirus, after a sample comes back positive. PCR tests that identify which specific variant a patient is carrying have been developed to assess positive samples for a variety of known strains. But because different variants possess similar mutations, definitive PCR tests are difficult to develop, and full genomic sequencing is a more reliable way to detect what variant is present in a particular sample.

The FDA does not currently authorize the use of any variant-specific tests for diagnostic use. Commercial and public health entities that process PCR testing and genomic sequencing for the purpose of variant identification are bound by patient privacy rules. Therefore, virtually everything we know about the presence of variants is at the public, not individual, level. This means that medical practitioners do not make treatment decisions based on the particular strain of the virus a patient has contracted. Rather, an awareness of the variants circulating in a particular region can inform public health decisions at large.

Disease Modeling and Forecasting

Infectious disease models are critical planning tools for policymakers and healthcare providers. Officials use them to allocate resources, such as medical staff and supplies, forecast the spread or severity of a disease, and predict the effects and costs of different intervention options. Models can also be used to anticipate future outbreaks based on past experiences. Accurate models must incorporate what is known about the mechanics of the virus spread itself, how

---

[19] https://www.fda.gov/medical-devices/coronavirus-covid-19-and-medical-devic es/sars-cov-2-viral-mutations- impact-covid-19-tests.

[20] https://www.fda.gov/regulatory-information/search-fda-guidance-documents/policy-evaluat ing-impact-viral- mutations-covid-19-tests.

human behaviors adapt over the course of the pandemic, and, increasingly, how prevalent particular strains of the virus are in a given area.

Accurately and robustly incorporating variants into disease forecasting models would require an increased capacity for genomic surveillance and data sharing.[21] At the end of 2020, the United States ranked 28th in percentage of coronavirus samples sequenced to detect variants – up from 43rd at the end of 2020,[22] but still far behind many of our global peers.[23] Genetic sequencing data is currently shared and accessed by researchers primarily on GISAID, a nonprofit started to share avian flu data.[24] Federal investments in data aggregation tools are necessary to ensure researchers, public health officials, and the American public have reliable models and forecasts through this pandemic and beyond.

Federal Activities on Variants[25]

In 2014, the White House National Science and Technology Council (NSTC) chartered a new Pandemic Prediction and Forecasting Science and Technology Working Group to coordinate Federal outbreak prediction capabilities, including capabilities to predict variants. In late 2016, this Working Group issued a roadmap report, "Towards Epidemic Prediction: Federal Efforts and Opportunities in Outbreak Modeling."[26] It included a list of 14 high-level policy recommendations for a coordinated multi-agency effort provide for robust data and information sharing, stronger outbreak model development and decision support tools, and a "One Health" strategy for integrating scientific information from various sources to more effectively predict infectious disease outbreaks. The report also presented a table of various activities in infectious disease modeling being conducted across 11 different federal agencies, such as modeling of foreign animal disease activities being conducted by USDA's Animal and Plant Health Inspection Service (APHIS) and the Biosurveillance Ecosystem activities at DOE's Los Alamos National Laboratory.

---

[21] https://www.latimes.com/science/story/2021-02-07/how-the-u-s-plans-to-keep-tabs-on-the-coronavirus-variants- in-circulation-here.

[22] https://www.washingtonpost.com/world/2020/12/23/us-leads-world-coronavirus-cases-ranks-43rd-sequencing- check-variants/.

[23] https://covidcg.org/?tab=global_sequencing.

[24] https://www.gisaid.org/hcov19-variants/.

[25] https://www.nytimes.com/2021/04/14/health/coronavirus-testing-variants.html.

[26] towards_epidemic_prediction-federal_efforts_and_opportunities.pdf (archives.gov).

The ability to sequence the genome of a viral sample is critical to establishing what disease variant has led to a patient's infection. In May 2020, the CDC's Advanced Molecular Detection program established a new lab consortium called the SARS-CoV-2 Sequencing for Public Health Emergency Response, Epidemiology, and Surveillance, or SPHERES, dedicated to collaborating on and aggregating results from genome sequencing of viral samples. SPHERES convenes scientists and data contributions from state and local public health laboratories, clinical laboratories, universities, and the private sector. Its objectives include identifying resource needs across the country so that genome sequencing can be more widely deployed, but also championing principles of quick and open data sharing and the use of common data and analysis standards.[27]

In a January 21, 2021 Executive Order, President Biden proposed a new interagency National Center for Epidemic Forecasting and Outbreak Analytics, which would support global efforts to prevent, detect, respond to, and recover from emerging biological threats.[28] In January 2021, CDC introduced the National SARS-CoV-2 Strain Surveillance (NS3) program, which asked state laboratories to remit viral sample data to CDC on a weekly basis in order to help establish a national picture of how variants are spreading and affecting patients.[29] On April 16, the Administration announced that the CDC will allocate $1.7 billion to states to scale up science capabilities for tracking and monitoring COVID-19 variants.[30]

Statement by Representative Bill Foster, Chairman, Subcommittee on Investigations and Oversight, Committee on Science, Space, and Technology, U.S. House of Representatives

Chairman FOSTER. This hearing will now come to order. Without objection, the Chair is authorized to declare a recess at any time. Before I deliver my opening remarks, I wanted to note the circumstances under which we're

---

[27] SPHERES | CDC.

[28] The White House, *National Security Memorandum on United States Global Leadership to Strengthen the International COVID-19Response and to Advance Global Health Security and Biological Preparedness.*

[29] FEB 2021 Revised NS3 FAQ_02052021 FNL.pdf (aphl.org).

[30] https://www.whitehouse.gov/briefing-room/statements-releases/2021/04/16/fact-sheet-biden-administration- announces-1-7-billion-investment-to-fight-covid-19-variants/.

meeting today. Pursuant to House Resolution 8, the Subcommittee is meeting virtually, and a couple of reminders for the Members about the conduct of this remote hearing. First, Members should keep their video feed on as long as they are present in the hearing. Members are responsible for their own microphones. Please also keep your microphones muted unless you're speaking. Finally, if Members have documents they wish to submit for the record, please email them to the Committee Clerk, whose email address was circulated prior to the hearing.

Well, good morning, and welcome to our Members and our panelists. Thank you for joining us for this hearing on COVID–19 variants. Over a year into the pandemic, we're all accustomed to a new normal: social distancing, mask wearing, and, of course, the virtual proceedings we're conducting today. Almost 60 percent of Americans have received at least one vaccination dose, and our ability to detect and monitor the spread of the virus puts us in a much better position than we were just one year ago.

But just as we've adapted to life in the pandemic, the virus has mutated as it continues to spread around the globe. Each new variant brings the potential for increased contagiousness, disease severity, and evasion of safety measures and vaccine-induced natural immunity. Today, most of the new variants seem to have evolved from national—natural evolutionary pressure, natural selection for infectiousness. One of the commonly expressed worries is about an escape variant of the virus, a superbug that is resistant to our vaccines and may—might evolve in a partially vaccinated population. In a worst-case scenario, such a variant would require us to start over from zero in our vaccine manufacturing, tests, and deployment.

One important policy decision that the United States faces is whether to hold in reserve vaccine manufacturing capacity for such a contingency or perhaps simply to reserve vaccine manufacturing capacity for possible booster shots, which may be required due to the waning of our immune response. This decision will be especially fraught if we conclude that we must use our manufacturing capacity to make booster shots for the U.S. at a time when the rest of the world may not be fully vaccinated.

To make those decisions, and many others, we need to evaluate the probability that new variants or escape variants, as well as what is known about the waning of our immune response from the vaccines, to the standard variants of the virus.

And, more broadly, we must ensure that the tools we use to detect, treat, and forecast the virus are keeping up with the emerging variants. Researchers, medical practitioners, and public health authorities have spent the last year standing up an unbelievably impressive network of testing, surveillance, treatment, and prevention tools. Thinking back to March 2020, it was unimaginable to many that by May 2021, more than half of Americans would be vaccinated against a virus that had just reached our shores. Disease monitoring tools require an unprecedented scale of data sharing and aggregation on an international level.

And, as the death rate in our country has been dropping for months, thanks to a better awareness of how to treat this disease, we must not lose any of the gains as this virus mutates, potentially increasing in contagiousness, severity, or its ability to escape our vaccines. It's important that we in the Federal Government support the efforts of researchers and public health agencies in conducting top-of-the-line research to inform health-protective policies.

Our witnesses here today will tell us about some of the amazing science that has come out of the work on the pandemic, and how we can best support their work now and into the future. The U.S. scientific enterprise has historically been equipped to answer those questions, and the Federal Government must continue to support and amplify this support.

In this fight, we must not lose sight of our Nation's place as a world leader and the importance of international collaboration. We have all seen the recent devastating news coming out of India, making this hearing all the more timely. Stories of overloaded hospitals, insufficient vaccine supplies, and mounting deaths. The more the virus spreads, the more mutations will occur, meaning more strains of virus will develop. No country is out of the woods until every country has the ability to reach herd immunity, or to paraphrase Dr. Rev. Martin Luther King, coronavirus anywhere is a threat to health everywhere.

The Biden Administration has committed to this global fight by rejoining the World Health Organization and the COVAX (COVID- 19 Vaccines Global Access) program, pledging $2 billion to support vaccine access in low- and middle-income countries. The United States is also sending 60 million doses of the AstraZeneca (AZ) vaccine overseas, but we must do more. All approved vaccines have shown to be efficacious in preventing severe forms of known variants, a triumph worth celebrating and something that we cannot take for granted into the future. Bolstering worldwide vaccine access must go hand-in-hand with continuing monitoring of vaccine efficacy in the face of new variants.

I look forward to hearing from our witnesses today about how we can best support the research that we need to end this pandemic and to prepare for the next.

[The prepared statement of Chairman Foster follows:]

Written Statement by Representative Bill Foster, Chairman, Subcommittee on Investigations and Oversight, Committee on Science, Space and Technology, U.S. House of Representatives

Good morning, and welcome to our members and our panelists. Thank you for joining us for this hearing on COVID–19 variants. Over a year into the pandemic, we're all accustomed to a new normal—social distancing, mask wearing, hand sanitizing, and, of course, the virtual proceedings we're conducting today. Almost 60 percent of Americans have received at least one vaccination dose, and our ability to detect and monitor the spread of the virus puts us in a much better position than we were just one year ago. But just as we've adapted to life in a pandemic, the virus has mutated as it continues to spread around the globe. Each new variant brings the potential for increased contagiousness, disease severity, and evasion of safety measures and vaccine-induced and natural immunity. We must ensure that the tools we use to detect, treat, and forecast the virus are keeping up with emerging variants.

Researchers, medical practitioners, and public health authorities have spent the last year standing up an unbelievably impressive network of testing, surveillance, treatment, and prevention tools. Thinking back to March 2020, it was unimaginable to many that by May 2021, more than half of Americans would be vaccinated against a virus that had just reached our shores. Disease monitoring tools require an unprecedented scale of data sharing and aggregation on an international level. And the death rate in our country has been dropping for months, thanks in part to a better awareness of how to treat this disease. We must not lose any of thesegains as the virus mutates, potentially increasing its contagiousness and severity. It is imperative that we in the federal government support the efforts of researchers and public health agencies in conducting top-of-the-line research to inform health- protective policies.

Our witnesses here today will tell us about some of the amazing science that has come out of the pandemic, and how we can best support their work. Each time a new variant pops up on the CDC website, I'm sure we all have the same questions. How effective are existing tests and vaccines? How will masking and distancing guidelines be adjusted based on the contagiousness of this new strain? Will the virus cause more severe illness that requires different treatments? The U.S. scientific enterprise is equipped to answer these questions, and the federal government must continue to support and amplify this work.

In this fight, we must not lose sight of our nation's place as a world leader and the importance of international collaboration. We have all seen the recent devastating news coming out of India, making this hearing all the more timely. Stories of overloaded hospitals, insufficient vaccine supplies, and mounting deaths. The more the virus spreads, the more mutations will occur, meaning more strains of the virus will develop. No country is out of the woods until every country has the ability to reach herd immunity. The Biden Administration has committed to this global fight by rejoining the World Health Organization and the COVAX program, pledging $2 billion to support vaccine access in low- and middle-income countries. The United States is also sending 60 million doses of the AstraZeneca vaccine overseas. All approved vaccines have shown to be efficacious in preventing severe disease from known variants—a triumph worth celebrating, and something we cannot take for granted. Bolstering worldwide vaccine access must go hand-in-hand with continued monitoring of vaccine efficacy in the face of new variants.

I look forward to hearing from our witnesses today about how we can best support the research we need to end this pandemic and prepare for the next.

I now yield to Ranking Member Obernolte for his remarks.

Statement by Representative Jay Obernolte, Ranking Member, Subcommittee on Investigations and Oversight, Committee on Science, Space, and Technology, U.S. House of Representatives

Chairman FOSTER. And I'll recognize my Ranking Member, Mr. Obernolte, for his—an opening statement.

Mr. OBERNOLTE. Thank you very much, Chairman Foster, and thank you for convening this very timely hearing on a very important topic. I am looking forward to hearing from our witnesses, and I'm particularly excited about this hearing because it gives us the opportunity to highlight the incredibly important role that our research community has had in fighting this epidemic. I believe that many of our Federal researchers are the unsung heroes of this epidemic, and I also believe that the development and deployment of the vaccines that have been accomplished in the last few months will go down as one of the greatest scientific achievements of mankind so far. So it can't be understated the incredible role that our research community has had in combatting this virus.

Unfortunately, though, it's clear that much more work needs to be done. If we look at the emergence of the different variants of COVID–19, it's clear that we need to invest more in research and development so that we understand a lot of the questions that are still unanswered, for example, the way that these variants emerge, whether or not these variants cause more or less severe illnesses, whether or not they're more or less transmissible, and the way that those variants respond to the various vaccines that have been developed and the way that we can develop vaccines in the future that anticipate those variants. So it's very important that we continue this investment in research into not only human biology but epidemiology and the spread of these variants.

I also want to highlight the important role that Congress has to play in stimulating this kind of research. The Federal Government is a natural—actually absolutely critical source of funding and of focusing attention on these efforts, and we need to continue that investment. I know that the Science, Space, and Technology Committee is considering a number of different bills that will continue that investment, and I fully support those efforts. I want to highlight one in particular, H.R. 2153, the Securing American Leadership in Science and Technology Act, which authorizes Department of Energy (DOE) infectious disease research program. I think that that's incredibly important, and I hope that that's something that's going to get attention in this Committee.

So, Mr. Chairman, thank you very much again for convening the hearing, and I'm looking forward to hearing from our witnesses.

[The prepared statement of Mr. Obernolte follows:]

Written Statement by Representative Jay Obernolte, Ranking Member, Subcommittee on Investigations and Oversight, Committee on Science, Space, and Technology, U.S. House of Representatives

Thank you, Chairman Foster, for holding today's important and timely hearing. I would also like to thank our expert witnesses for their participation today.

I look forward to learning more about the important contributions the Department of Energy (DOE) Office of Science's National Laboratories are making to combat the COVID–19 virus, and what role they can play moving forward to combat other infectious diseases. Thank you, Dr. Streiffer for being here today and for all the important work you do at Argonne National Laboratory.

Our nation's research enterprise has demonstrated it has the expertise, resources, and talent to fight this pandemic. We have supercomputers, advanced manufacturing techniques, and even advanced photon sources being used to fight COVID– 19.

The DOE National Labs have a history of using technical solutions to respond to national and international emergencies, and when the COVID–19 pandemic hit, the labs were prepared, ready, and willing to serve on the front lines. DOE received $99.5M in the *CARES Act* to fund research at the National Labs to better understand COVID–19. This funding has since been fully expended.

At the start of the pandemic, DOE pivoted and launched the National Virtual Biotechnical Laboratory (NVBL) to mobilize the resources of the Department of Energy's 17 National Labs to engage in critical COVID–19 research. Projects within NVBL are focused on molecular design for medical therapeutics, development and evaluation of COVID–19 testing, epidemiological and transpiration modeling, and advanced manufacturing.

I would also like to highlight that decades of investment in basic scientific research involving the National Labs contributed to the unprecedented speed COVID–19 vaccines were developed and distributed. These investments have been truly life- saving.

The accomplishments made possible through the NVBL demonstrate the power of the U.S. innovation ecosystem, when you have DOE National labs, universities, and companies all working together to address a national and societal challenge.

As the original COVID–19 virus and new variants continue to spread across the globe, it is imperative that the United States continues to make critical investments in basic research for the health and safety of our nation. To date, the Centers for Disease Control and Prevention (CDC) have identified five COVID–19 Variants of Concern (VOCs) in the United States. Researchers are paying close attention to these VOCs as according to the CDC, they appear to spread more easily and quickly than other identified Variants of Interest (VOIs).

There remains a lot of information public health officials and researchers do not yet know about COVID–19 variants, and further studies are needed. For example, researchers still need to learn how easily emerging COVID–19 variants spread, if they cause milder or more severe illness, if they are detected by currently available viral tests, if they respond to medications currently being used to treat COVID–19, and whether existing authorized vaccines protect people from them. The DOE National Labs can build upon previous COVID–19 research work and get ahead in the race against COVID–19 mutations. The National Labs have existing infrastructure, resources, and experts ready to deploy, and can continue to play a leading role in addressing key concerns and challenges to confront the COVID–19 pandemic and beyond.

Before I close, I would like to highlight H.R. 2153, the Securing American Leadership in *Science and Technology Act (SALSTA)*, which was introduced by Full Committee Ranking Member Lucas in March, and which I am an original cosponsor of. This legislation includes an authorization for a DOE emerging infectious disease research program and high-performance computing research consortium.

I hope that today's hearing will con tinue an important dialogue on the role of Federal science agencies in supporting R&D to combat the COVID–19 virus and propose new and innovative solutions for infectious disease responses in the future.

Thank you, and I yield back.

Statement by Representative Eddie Bernice Johnson, Chairwoman, Committee on Science, Space, and Technology, U.S. House of Representatives

Chairman FOSTER. Thank you. And we are honored to have the Full Committee Chairwoman, Ms. Johnson, with us today, and the Chair now recognizes the Chairwoman for an opening statement. Chairwoman JOHNSON. Well, thank you very much, and good morning. Let me thank you for holding this hearing today and thank all of our witnesses for joining us this morning. Dr. Abdool Karim, I understand you are halfway around the world right now, so good evening to you.

Today's hearing could not be more timely. The United States has already made incredible strides in making safe, accessible vaccines available to all adults. Just this week, the FDA (Food and Drug Administration) extended an authorization for 12- to 15-year-olds to receive the Pfizer vaccine. And I understand that some of our basic science research was performed at one of our national laboratories, the home of one of our witness's laboratory. These scientific achievements were a gift to the world, and they've already saved millions of lives, and they will save millions more.

In the United States, every teenager and adult now has access to the tools they need to protect themselves and loved ones. We must not squander this gift. We have no time to waste because viral variants are threatening the progress the United States has made toward defeating COVID–19. In recent weeks, one variant has brought the entire nation of India to its knees. And the longer the COVID–19 persists around the globe, the more mutations will emerge. Pandemics know no borders. An emerging variant anywhere is a public health threat everywhere, as you have said, Mr. Chair.

Our witnesses today will help us understand how emerging variants make it even more urgent to vaccinate fast, not just in the United States, but across the globe. I also look forward to hearing about the scientific tools we can use to spot a variant. The Federal Government supports an impressive range of infectious diseases— disease modeling, data sharing, and surveillance activities. We know now that these programs should have been coordinating more closely before the pandemic. A 2016 White House report offered a roadmap for exactly that: stitching together science activities across a dozen different agencies to enable better models of how diseases spread and change. Unfortunately, we did not get far enough on implementing these recommendations before COVID–19 reached our shores.

But it isn't too late to continue to improve the Federal approach to disease forecasting and surveillance for this present-day crisis. We can deploy our best Federal science capabilities to detect and understand variants as early as possible. This helps public officials and healthcare providers have the quality information they need to protect and save lives.

Thank you, Subcommittee Chairman Foster and Ranking Member, for putting together this timely discussion, and I yield back.

[The prepared statement of Chairwoman Johnson follows (next page):]

Written Statement by Representative Eddie Bernice Johnson, Chairwoman, Committee on Science, Space, and Technology, U.S. House of Representatives

Good morning and thank you to our witnesses for joining us this morning. Dr. Abdool Karim, I understand you are halfway around the world right now, so good evening to you.

Today's hearing could not be more timely. The United States has already made incredible strides in making safe, accessible vaccines available to all adults. Just this week, the FDA extended an authorization for 12- to 15-year-olds to receive the Pfizer vaccine. I understand that some of the basic science research performed at Argonne National Laboratory, home to one of our witnesses today, was a foundational part of creating mRNA vaccines. These scientific achievements were a gift to the world. They have already saved millions of lives, and they will save millions more. In the United States, every teenager and adult now has access to the tools they need to protect ourselves and our loved ones.

But we must not squander this gift.

We have no time to waste, because viral variants are threatening the progress the United States has made toward defeating COVID–19. In recent weeks, one variant has brought the entire nation of India to its knees. And the longer COVID–19 persists around the globe, the more mutations will emerge. Pandemics know no borders; an emerging variant anywhere is a public health threat everywhere. Our witnesses today will help us understand how emerging variants make it even more urgent to vaccinate fast—not in just the United States, but across the globe.

I also look forward to hearing about all the scientific tools we can use to spot a variant. The federal government supports an impressive range of infectious disease modeling, data sharing, and surveillance activities. We know now that these programs should have been coordinating more closely before the pandemic. A 2016 White House report offered a roadmap for exactly this: stitching together science activities across a dozen different agencies to enable better models of how diseases spread and change. Unfortunately, we did not get far enough on implementing those recommendations before COVID–19 reached our shores.

But it isn't too late to continue to improve the federal approach to disease forecasting and surveillance for this present-day crisis. We can deploy our best federal science capabilities to detect and understand variants as early as possible. This helps public officials and healthcare providers have the quality information they need to protect the public and save lives.

Thank you Subcommittee Chairman Foster and Ranking Member Obernolte for putting together this timely discussion. I yield back.

***

Chairman FOSTER. Thank you. And if there are any Members who wish to submit additional opening statements, your statements will be added to the record at this point.

At this time, I'd like to introduce our witnesses. Our first witness is Dr. Salim Abdool Karim. Dr. Abdool Karim is a clinical infectious disease epidemiologist who has played a leading role in the global COVID–19 pandemic response. He is Director for the Center for AIDS—the AIDS Programme of Research in South Africa, CAPRISA, and CAPRISA Professor of Global Health at Columbia University. Dr. Abdool Karim is also one of the nine members of the World Health Organization's Science Council. His contributions during the pandemic have focused on the epidemiology of SARS- CoV–2 variants, including their impact on vaccine and natural immunity.

Next is Dr. Nathan Grubaugh, Associate Professor of Epidemiology at the Yale School of Public Health and head of the Grubaugh Lab where he studies virus emergence, transmission, and evolution. During disease outbreaks, his lab sequences viruses for epidemiological investigations, determines the disease phenotype and transmission fitness of novel virus mutations, and maps the evolutionary pathways that a virus may take to adapt.

Our third witness is Dr. Stephen Streiffer. Dr. Streiffer hold several positions at Argonne National Laboratory in the Illinois 11th District I might add, including Deputy Laboratory Director for Science and Technology. He is one of the founding Co-Chairs of the National Virtual Biotechnology Laboratory, or NVBL, a consortium of DOE national labs founded to address the COVID–19 crisis. The NVBL has used their scientific and technical expertise to address medical supply shortages, discover potential drugs to fight the virus, develop and verify COVID–19 testing methods, model disease spread and impact across the Nation, and understand virus transport in buildings and in the environment.

Our final witness is Dr. Caitlin Rivers, Senior Scholar at the Johns Hopkins Center for Health Security and an Assistant Professor in the Department of Environmental Health and Engineering at Johns Hopkins

Bloomberg School of Public Health. She's an epidemiologist specializing in emerging infectious diseases and has anchored or contributed to several reports on COVID–19 variants and the national pandemic strategy. Her research focuses broadly on improving public health preparedness and the response to large- scale events.

And, as our witnesses should know, you'll each have five minutes for your spoken testimony. Your written testimony will be included in the record for the hearing. And when you've all completed your spoken testimony, we will begin with questions and each Member will have five minutes to question the panel.

If time allows, we may have a second round of questioning. In addition, if there is interest in—among the Members at the close of the hearing, may—we may turn off the livestream and have an informal discussion with the panelists, something we do under normal circumstances and is possible also here.

We will now start with Dr. Abdool Karim, so you are now recognized for five minutes.

Statement of Dr. Salim Abdool Karim, Director of Caprisa

Dr. ABDOOL KARIM. Thank you very much, Chairman Johnson. It's indeed an honor for me to be here and provide some testimony. I submitted a slide set. I'm going to ask for that to be projected.

[Slide follows:]

SARS-CoV-2 variants: Implications for public health and the Covid-19 endgame

House Committee on Science, Space, and Technology, Subcommittee on Investigations & Oversight
Hearing on "*COVID-19 Variants and Evolving Research Needs*", May 12, 2021

Salim S. Abdool Karim, *FRS*

Director: CAPRISA – Center for the AIDS Program of Research in South Africa
CAPRISA Professor of Global Health, Mailman School of Public Health, Columbia University
Adjunct Professor in Immunology and Infectious Diseases, Harvard University
Adjunct Professor of Medicine: Cornell University
Pro Vice-Chancellor (Research): University of KwaZulu-Natal
Member: African Task Force for Coronavirus

COLUMBIA UNIVERSITY | MAILMAN SCHOOL of PUBLIC HEALTH

CAPRISA

Dr. ABDOOL KARIM. I speak to you from South Africa where I am based at—and the Nelson R. Mandela School of Medicine at an NIH- (National Institutes of Health-) funded research center. I'm actually at ground zero where one of the world's most concerning variants was first described. So I'm going to briefly touch on the variants. I want to talk about the implications for public health and the COVID–19 end game.

Next slide.[Slide follows:]

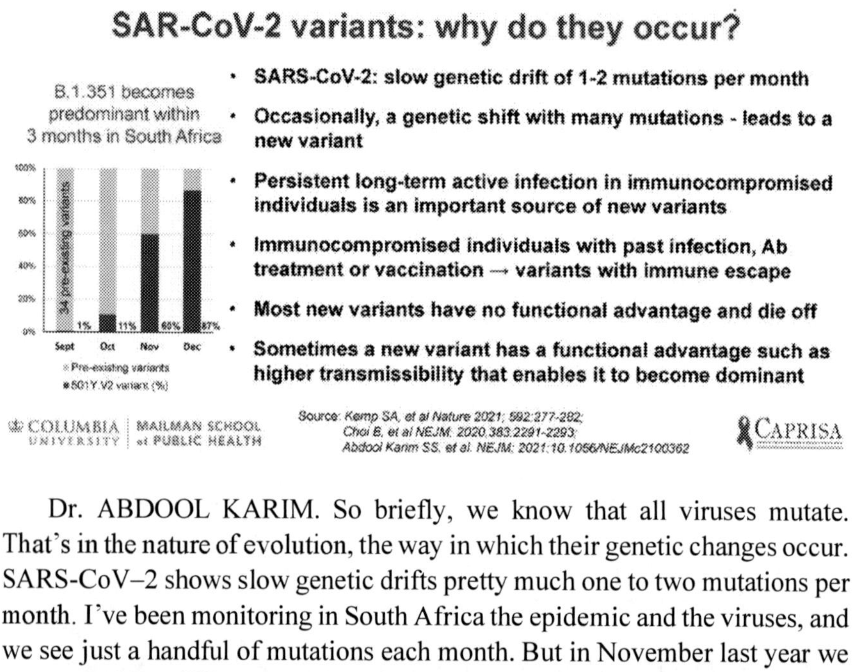

Dr. ABDOOL KARIM. So briefly, we know that all viruses mutate. That's in the nature of evolution, the way in which their genetic changes occur. SARS-CoV–2 shows slow genetic drifts pretty much one to two mutations per month. I've been monitoring in South Africa the epidemic and the viruses, and we see just a handful of mutations each month. But in November last year we saw something different, not just the slow antigenic drift but a shift, a major new mutant with 23 different mutations. And to give you some idea of its advantage and its functional advantage that it obtained, I point you to the graph on the left-hand side. Initially, in September, we had 34 pre-existing variants that were transmitted. The next month the new mutation referred to as B.1.351, constituted 11 percent of all the viruses. A month later, November, it was 60 percent, and by December, 87 percent of all the viruses transmitted were this new variant B.1.351.

Next slide, please.[Slide follows (next page):]

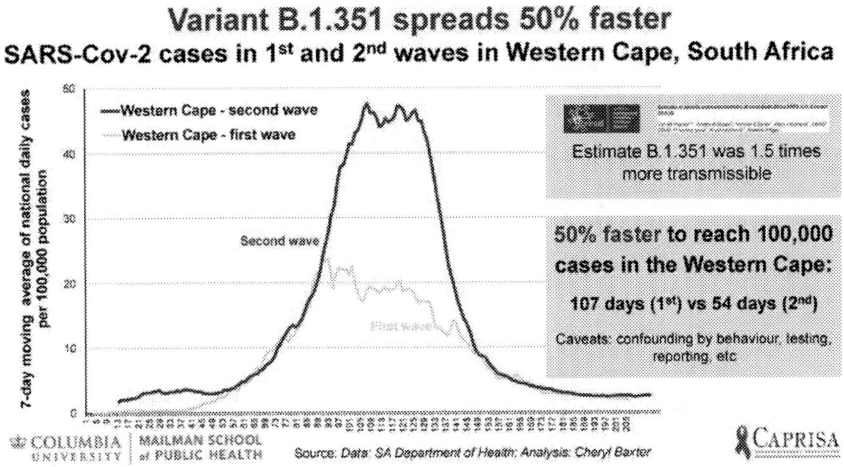

Dr. ABDOOL KARIM. And to give you some idea of what that has meant in comparing the first wave with pre-existing variants in the light yellow line you can see that the second wave, due to this new, more highly transmissible variant, the B.1.351 variant, is about 50 percent faster. If you just take one province in South Africa, Western Cape, it reached 100,000 cases within a matter of 54 days compared to the first wave where it took 107 days.

Next slide, please. [Slide follows:]

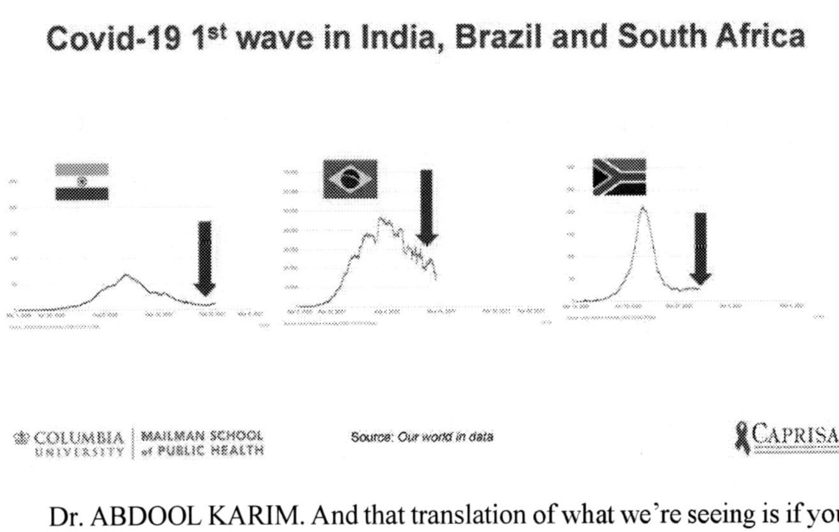

Dr. ABDOOL KARIM. And that translation of what we're seeing is if you take the three countries, India, Brazil, and South Africa, each of them in the first waves dealt with a pretty substantial wave, but what happened was as the epidemic settled, they all began to look at this epidemic in a different way.

Next slide. [Slide follows:]

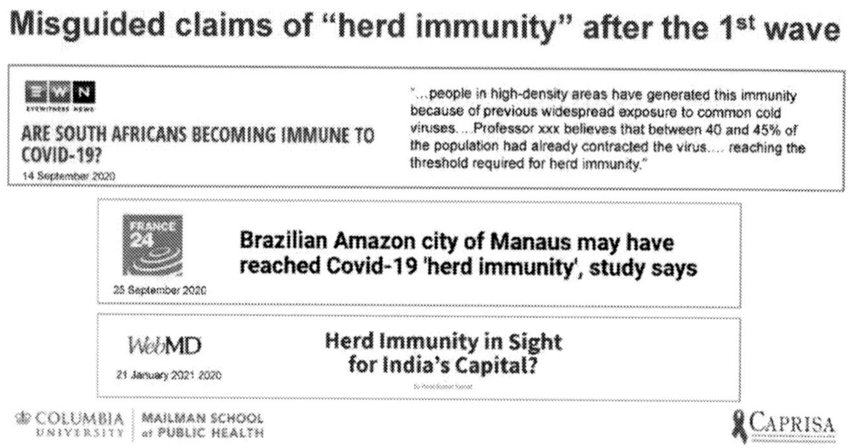

Dr. ABDOOL KARIM. And what we began to see was the—that each of these countries, they thought that they had conquered this virus. They had become immune, that they've developed some kind of protection from natural infection. We saw that in South Africa, we saw that in Brazil, we saw that in India.

Next slide.[Slide follows:]

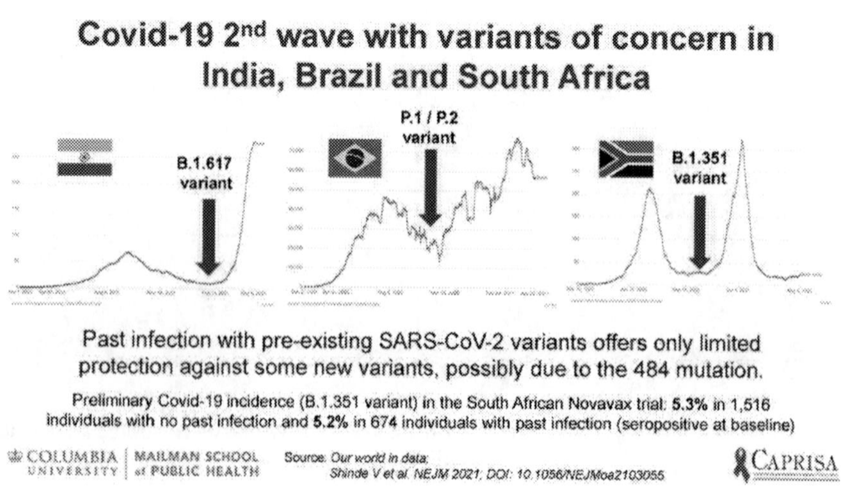

Dr. ABDOOL KARIM. And what happened was complacency that set in, and this is what happened. In each of those settings, a new variant. In India, the B.1.617; in Brazil, the P.1 and P.2 variants; and in South Africa, the B.1.351 variant. And in South Africa the data we have shows quite clearly at this point that the B.1.351 variant was able to escape immunity that was acquired in the first wave. And so what we are seeing is reinfections occurring quite commonly in South Africa.

Next slide, please. [Slide follows:]

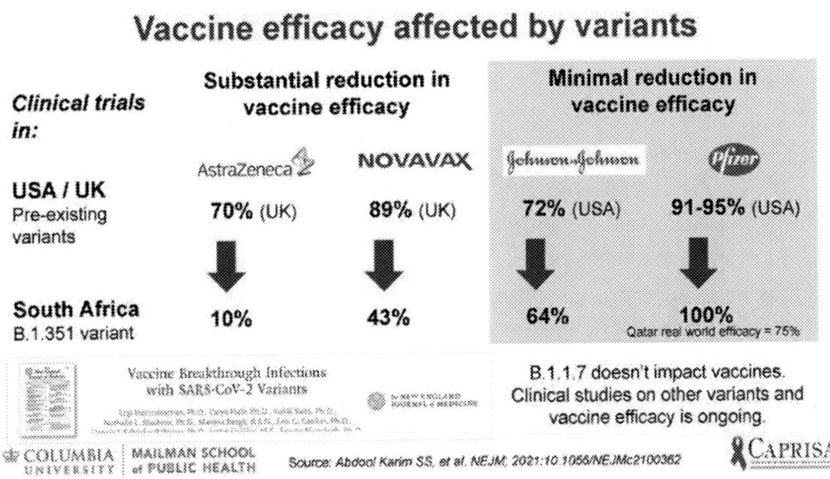

Dr. ABDOOL KARIM. So if we look at where we are in terms of vaccines, that is perhaps the most concerning of the things that we see and that if you take the AstraZeneca vaccine with 70 percent efficacious in the U.K. but only 10 percent efficacious in South Africa. Novavax, 89 percent but only 43 percent. And we are seeing breakthrough variants. Fortunately, vaccines like the Johnson & Johnson (J&J) and the Pfizer vaccine have maintained their efficacy.

Next slide. [Slide follows (next page):]

Conclusion

- Expect more variants! No country is safe until every country is safe
- Maximal viral suppression needed to prevent the emergence and spread of new variants overcoming immunity from vaccination or past infection
- No single action is going to be sufficient to prevent the spread of the virus: Public health measures must be maintained in tandem with vaccination
- Need to strengthen genomic surveillance in many countries as the situation may be even more severe than it appears at present
- Next generation vaccines to elicit broadly neutralizing antibodies currently being developed are expected to overcome immune escape by variants

COLUMBIA UNIVERSITY | MAILMAN SCHOOL of PUBLIC HEALTH CAPRISA

Dr. ABDOOL KARIM. And this is my last slide where I'll just make some parting comments that we should expect more variants, that no country is safe, as Chairman Johnson has pointed out so eloquently, until every country is safe, and that we need maximal suppression and that no single action is likely to be sufficient to prevent the spread of the virus. We're going to need our public health measures in addition to our vaccination programs. We need to strengthen genomic surveillance. And even though we are expecting next-generation vaccines to produce more broadly neutralizing antibodies and we expect they will impact on the escape variants, I suspect that we will continually see this virus finding ways to escape immunity.

Thank you very much, Chairman.

[The prepared statement of Dr. Abdool Karim follows:]

Written Statement of Dr. Salim Abdool Karim, Director of CAPRISA

Background

Currently there are multiple SARS-CoV-2 variants circulating across the world. These variants arise through natural variation, replication errors, cross-species transmission or immune pressure. Viruses with higher viral fitness and transmissibility are more likely to become dominant in the population. While most of variants are not a cause for concern, variants that acquire mutations in the functional parts of the virus, for example the receptor binding domain (RBD) of the spike protein, raise concerns. Accelerated changes leading tomultiple mutations in the infecting virus have been observed in immunocompromised patients with persistent SARS-CoV-2 infection.[31,32] In an immunosuppressed patient, who experienced persistent viral shedding over 154 days, the virus developed several geneticchanges, especially in the spike gene and the RBD.[31]

SARS-CoV-2 variants have been classified by the US Centers for Disease Control and Prevention (CDC) as variants of interest), variants of concern, and variants of high consequence. Until recently, there were three variants[33] that had rapidly become dominantwithin their countries that were classified as variants of concern; the B.1.1.7 (VOC- 202012/01), B.1.351 (501Y.V2) and P.1 (B.1.1.28.1).

The B.1.1.7 variant (23 mutations with 17 amino acid changes) was first described in the UKon 14 December 2020, the B.1.351 variant (23 mutations with 17 amino acid changes) was initially reported in South Africa on 18 December 2020 while the P.1 variant (about 35 mutations with 17 amino acid changes) was reported on 12 January 2021 from Brazil. By 5May 2021, the B.1.1.7, B.1.351 and P.1 variants have been reported in 114, 67 and 37 countries, respectively.[33] All three variants have the N501Y mutation that changes the aminoacid asparagine (N) to tyrosine (Y) at position 501 in the RBD of the spike protein. Both the B.1.351 and P.1 variants have two additional RBD mutations K417N/T and E484K. These mutations increase binding affinity of RBD to the Angiotensin-converting enzyme 2 (ACE-2)receptor ACE2.[34]

In March 2021, another new variant, the CAL.20C (B.1.427 & B.1.429) variant, which was originally reported in California, was classified as the fourth variant of concern. The varianthas one mutation in the RBD at position 452 (L452R) and 45% of current samples in California are this variant.

---

[31] Choi B, Choudhary MC, Regan J, et al. Persistence and Evolution of SARS-CoV-2 in an Immunocompromised Host. *N Eng J Med* 2020;383:2291-3.

[32] Kemp SA, Collier DA, Datir RP, et al. SARS-CoV-2 evolution during treatment of chronic infection. *Nature* 2021;592:277-82.

[33] Cov-lineages.org. *SARS-CoV-2 lineages - New variant report.* Available from: https://cov-lineages.org/global_report.html (accessed: 11 January 2021); 2021.

[34] Greaney AJ, Loes AN, Crawford KHD, et al. Comprehensive mapping of mutations to the SARS-CoV-2 receptor-binding domain that affect recognition by polyclonal human serum antibodies. *bioRxiv*, 2021. https://doi.org/10.1101/2020.12.31.425021.

There are also several variants of interest, including: B1.525, B1.526, B.1.617 and P.2. The B.1.525 variant, which carries some of the same mutations as B.1.1.7, and the B.1.526 which carries the E484K or S477N mutation, has been spreading in New York. The B.1.617is prevalent in India and carries the E484Q and L452R spike mutations, among its 13 other mutations. Emerging evidence from India suggests that B.1.617 spreads more rapidly andhad been reported from 28 countries by May 3, 2021.

The emergence of these new variants raise four key concerns, viz. their impact on a) viral transmissibility, b) disease severity, c) reinfection rates (escape from natural immunity) and d) vaccine effectiveness (escape from vaccine-induced immunity).

Transmissibility

The variants of concern spread more easily and quickly than other variants, which may lead to more cases of Covid-19 in a shorter period. The B.1.351 variant has been estimated to be 50%[35] more transmissible than pre-existing variants in South Africa, and B.1.1.7 to be between 43% and 82%[36] more transmissible than pre-existing variants in the UK. The P.1 variant is estimated to be about 2.5 times more transmissible than pre-existing variants,[37] while the B.1.427 and B.1.429 variants are about 20% more transmissible.[38]

Disease Severity

With regards to severity of the variants of concern, there is evidence in both directions. Hospital admission rates, clinical profile of admitted patients and hospital case fatality rates were similar in the first and second waves in South

---

[35] Pearson CAB, Russell TMR, Davies NG, et al. Estimates of severity and transmissibility of novelSouth Africa SARS-CoV-2 variant 501Y.V2. *CMMID Repository*, 2021. https://cmmid.github.io/topics/covid19/sa-novel-variant.html.

[36] Davies N, Barnard RC, Jarvis CI, et al. Estimated transmissibility and severity of novel SARS-CoV-2 Variant of Concern 202012/01 in England. *CMMID Repository*, 2020. https://cmmid.github.io/topics/covid19/uk-novel-variant.html.

[37] Coutinho RM, Marquitti FMD, Ferreira LS, et al. Model-based evaluation of transmissibility and reinfection for the P.1 variant of the SARS-CoV-2. *medRxiv*, 2021:2021.03.03.21252706.

[38] Deng X, Garcia-Knight MA, Khalid MM, et al. Transmission, infectivity, and antibody neutralization of an emerging SARS-CoV-2 variant in California carrying a L452R spike proteinmutation. *medRxiv* 2021:2021.03.07.21252647.

Africa. However, emerging evidence from the UK indicates that B.1.1.7 may be associated with an increased risk of death compared to pre-existing variants in the UK.[39] The variants may also indirectly increase mortality through their greater transmissibility, which rapidly overburdens health services, compromising access to, and quality of, hospital care. While there is no evidence that antivirals and anti-inflammatory treatments are affected, treatment with convalescent serum and monoclonal antibodies may no longer be effective.[40,41,42]

Escape from Natural Immunity

With regard to escape from natural immunity, the B.1.1.7 variant showed a modest decrease in neutralization activity, by a factor of 1.5, whereas the B.1.351 variant showed complete escape from neutralizing antibodies in 48% of convalescent serum samples (21 of 44) obtained from patients who had previously had Covid-19.[43]A serendipitous finding from a vaccine trial in South Africa, in which 30% of the enrolled participants had previously been infected with SARS-CoV-2, was that the incidence of Covid-19, as confirmed on polymerase chain reaction, was 5.3% among seronegative enrollees and 5.2% among seropositive enrollees in the placebo group after 60 days of follow-up.[44] The P.1 variants also has reduced neutralization by convalescent sera.[45] For the B.1.427 and B.1.429 variants, antibody neutralization assays

---

[39] Horby P, Huntley C, Davies N, et al. NERVTAG paper on COVID-19 variant of concern B.1.1.7. Available from: https://www.gov.uk/government/publications/nervtag-paper-on-covid-19-variant- of-concern-b117: SAGE meeting report; 2021.

[40] Wibmer CK, Ayres F, Hermanus T, et al. SARS-CoV-2 501Y.V2 escapes neutralization by SouthAfrican COVID-19 donor plasma. *bioRxiv: the preprint server for biology*, 2021:doi: https://doi.org/ 10.1101/2021.01.18.427166.

[41] Shen X, Tang H, McDanal C, et al. SARS-CoV-2 variant B.1.1.7 is susceptible to neutralizing antibodies elicited by ancestral Spike vaccines. *bioRxiv : the preprint server for biology*, 2021:2021.01.27.428516.

[42] Wang P, Casner RG, Nair MS, et al. Increased Resistance of SARS-CoV-2 Variant P.1 to Antibody Neutralization. *bioRxiv : the preprint server for biology*, 2021:2021.03.01.433466.

[43] Wibmer CK, Ayres F, Hermanus T, et al. SARS-CoV-2 501Y.V2 escapes neutralization by SouthAfrican COVID-19 donor plasma. *Nature Medicine*, 2021.

[44] Shinde V, Bhikha S, Hoosain Z, et al. Efficacy of NVX-CoV2373 Covid-19 Vaccine against the B.1.351 Variant. *N Engl J Med*, 2021:10.1056/NEJMoa2103055.

[45] Wang P, Casner RG, Nair MS, et al. Increased resistance of SARS-CoV-2 variant P.1 to antibody neutralization. *Cell Host Microbe*, 2021.

showed 4.0 to 6.7-fold decreases in neutralizing titres from convalescent patients.[46]

Escape from Vaccine-Induced Immunity

Regarding escape from vaccine-induced immunity, the B.1.1.7, B.1.427 and B.1.429 variantsshowed modest decreases in neutralizing activity in serum samples obtained from vaccinated persons.[11,16,47,48] The serum neutralizing activity for the B.1.351 variant among vaccinated persons was lower by a factor of 1.6 to 8.6 for the BBIBP-CorV vaccine[4919], the BNT162b2 vaccine[17], and the mRNA-1273 vaccine[5020] but was lower by a factor of up to 86, including complete immune escape, for the AZD1222 vaccine.[51,52] Neutralizing activity for the P.1 variant among vaccinated persons was lower by a factor of 6.7 for the BNT162b2 vaccine[53] and by a factor of 4.5 for the mRNA-1273 vaccine. The clinical relevance of the lower neutralization activity for either mild or severe Covid-19 is not clear. Efficacy in clinical trials was substantially lower for two of the four vaccines tested during transmission of the B.1.351 variant in South Africa than efficacy in trials conducted in countries with pre-existing variants.

---

[46] Deng X, Garcia-Knight MA, Khalid MM, et al. Transmission, infectivity, and antibody neutralization of an emerging SARS-CoV-2 variant in California carrying a L452R spike proteinmutation. *medRxiv*, 2021.

[47] Wang P, Liu L, Iketani S, et al. Increased Resistance of SARS-CoV-2 Variants B.1.351 and B.1.1.7 to Antibody Neutralization. *bioRxiv: the preprint server for biology*, 2021:2021. 01.25.428137.

[48] Polack FP, Thomas SJ, Kitchin N, et al. Safety and Efficacy of the BNT162b2 mRNA Covid-19Vaccine. *N Eng J Med*, 2020;383:2603-15.

[49] Huang B, Dai L, Wang H, et al. Neutralization of SARS-CoV-2 VARIANTS OF CONCERN 501Y.V2 by human antisera elicited by both inactivated BBIBP-CorV and recombinant dimeric RBD ZF2001 vaccines. *bioRxiv: the preprint server for biology* 2021:https:// doi.org/10.1101/2021.02. 01.429069.

[50] Wu K, Werner AP, Moliva JI, et al. mRNA-1273 vaccine induces neutralizing antibodies againstspike mutants from global SARS-CoV-2 variants. *bioRxiv: the preprint server for biology*, 2021.

[51] Madhi SA, Baillie V, Cutland CL, et al. Efficacy of the ChAdOx1 nCoV-19 Covid-19 Vaccine against the B.1.351 Variant. *N Eng J Med*, 2021: 10.1056/NEJMoa2102214.

[52] Voysey M, Clemens SAC, Madhi SA, et al. Safety and efficacy of the ChAdOx1 nCoV-19 vaccine (AZD1222) against SARS-CoV-2: an interim analysis of four randomised controlled trials in Brazil, South Africa, and the UK. *Lancet*, 2021;397:99-111.

[53] Garcia-Beltran WF, Lam EC, St. Denis K, et al. Multiple SARS-CoV-2 variants escape neutralization by vaccine-induced humoral immunity. *Cell*, 2021. doi: https://doi.org/ 10.1016/ j.cell.2021.03.013.

Responses to Questions from the Committee

1. What is the state of data sharing among countries regarding variants developing and spreading across the globe?

There are a few different databases being used to load SAR-CoV-2 sequences onto the internet. The most widely used is a database known as GISAID. Since January 2020, more than 1.5 million SARS-CoV-2 sequences have been included in GISAID. Of the 93 countries that have had more than 100,000 Covid-19 cases, 19 countries have contributed more than 1% of their viral sequences, with 5 countries (Norway, Denmark, Japan, Switzerland and the UK) contributing more than 5% of their viral sequences.

GISAID doesn't allow sequences to be reshared publicly without due acknowledgement to the original source.[54] While some researchers have regarded the GISAID processes of acknowledgement of sequence source as a hindrance, others consider it to be important acknowledgement of the scientific contributions of those who have provided the sequences. Other databases that also provide sequences on the internet such as the European Nucleotide Archive (ENA) and the NIH's the National Center for Biotechnology Information (NCBI) do not require acknowledgement of those who provided the original sequence. There are also websites that summarize data from these databases, such as https://outbreak.info, https://covariants.org and https://cov-spectrum.ethz.ch.

Researchers across the globe have free access to SARS-CoV-2 sequences from any of the databases providing genetic sequences on the internet. These databases are very widely used and provide a valuable repository for global information on the viruses; an essential requirement for future vaccine development.

2. Are existing vaccines efficacious in reducing the spread of known COVID-19 variants?

Some vaccines are highly effective against the variants of concern. For example, the efficacy of the Johnson & Johnson (J&J) vaccine was consistent across multiple variants including two variants of concern. It was 72% efficacious in the US (n = 17,793; D614G variant), 68% efficacious in Brazil

[54] van Noorden R. Scientists call for fully open sharing of coronavirus genome data. *Nature,* 2021;590, :195-6.

(n = 6,666; P.2 variant) and 64% efficacious in South Africa (n = 4,912; B.1.351 variant).[55] Similarly, the Pfizer–BioNTech vaccine, which was shown to be > 90% effective against pre-existing variants, has been shown in a study in South Africa to also be > 90% effective against the B.1.351 variant.[56] Data from Qatar, which implemented a large- scale vaccination programme in the presence of the B.1.1.7 and B.1.351 variants shows that the Pfizer–BioNTech vaccine was 90% effective against the B.1.1.7 variant and 75% effective against the B.1.351 variant 27. Further, the Pfizer–BioNTech vaccine effectiveness in Qatar against the B.1.1.7 and B.1.351 variants for severe, critical, or fatal disease was very high, at 97.4%.[57]

On the other hand, some vaccines have reduced efficacy in the presence of variants of concern. The efficacy of the AstraZeneca vaccine 70% in the UK (D614G variant) but only 10% efficacious against the B.1.351 variant in South Africa.[58,59] Similarly, the Novavax vaccine was only half as efficacious against the B.1.351 variant as it was 89% efficacious in the UK compared to 43% in South Africa14. Unfortunately, the South African studies of the AstraZeneca and Novovax vaccines predominantly included young people and so had no cases of severe disease. Hence, there is no clinical evidence on whether these vaccines that have minimal, if any, efficacy for mild / moderate disease due to the B.1.351 variant of concern have any efficacy for severe disease. Some speculate, drawing upon indirect evidence, that even though some of the vaccines such as AstraZeneca are not effective in preventing asymptomatic, mild or moderate infections due to B.1.351, they may still prevent severe disease from B.1.351 infections, there is no clinical evidence for this conclusion.

---

[55] Sadoff J, Gray G, Vandebosch A, et al. Safety and Efficacy of Single-Dose Ad26.COV2.S Vaccine against Covid-19. *N Eng J Med*, 2021.

[56] Pfizer. Pfizer and Biotech confirm high efficacy and no serious safety concerns through up to sixmonths following second dose in updated topline analysis of landmark Covid-19 vaccine study.Available from: https://www.pfizer.com/news/press-release/press-release-detail/ pfizer-and- biontech-confirm-high-efficacy-and-no-serious. Accessed: 5 May 2021; 2021.

[57] Abu-Raddad LJ, Chemaitelly H, Butt AA. Effectiveness of the BNT162b2 Covid-19 Vaccine against the B.1.1.7 and B.1.351 Variants. *N Eng J Med*, 2021:10.1056/NEJMc2104974.

[58] Madhi SA, Baillie V, Cutland CL, et al. Efficacy of the ChAdOx1 nCoV-19 Covid-19 Vaccine against the B.1.351 Variant. *N Engl J Med*, 2021:10.1056/NEJMoa2102214.

[59] Voysey M, Sue Ann Costa Clemens SAC, Madhi SA, et al. Single dose administration, and the influence of the timing of the booster dose on immunogenicity and efficacy of ChAdOx1 nCoV-19(AZD1222) vaccine. *Lancet*, pre-print, 2020:https://papers.ssrn.com/sol3/papers.cfm?abstract_id=3777268.

3. What role do vaccines play in reducing the spread of existing variants and the emergence of new variants?

The vaccines play a critical role in suppressing viral replication which in turn reduces the risk of emergence of variants. However, the use of vaccines creates immune pressure on the virus, especially if there is persistent viral replication. In immunocompromised individuals there is the risk of new variants emerging.[2] If these immunocompromised individuals were vaccinated or received monoclonal antibody treatments, their persistent viral replication may lead to immune escape mutations. If such mutations enhance escape from vaccine-induced immunity, the vaccines would be rendered less effective.

The Covid-19 pandemic has illustrated that no single action is sufficient to prevent the spread of the virus. Strong public health measures against the virus must be maintained in tandem with global vaccination programs to achieve the goal of maximum suppression (see Lancet commission on Covid-19 report "SARS-CoV-2 variants: the need for urgent public health action beyond vaccines" - Annexure 1).

For viruses to succeed in spreading in a highly vaccinated population, they would need to evade vaccine-induced immunity. The current variants with predominant mutations in the receptor binding domain at positions 501, 484, 417 and 452 predate widespread availability of vaccines as most originated between October and December 2020. Over the coming months we can reasonably expect new variants to emerge that are able to escape vaccine-induced immunity because the virus is being put under pressure from widescale vaccination at present. This creates a catch-22 situation; when vaccinations are being scaled-up while viral transmission is high, as is occurring in the US and Brazil, SARS-CoV-2 has a higher likelihood of acquiring escape mutations potentially undermining the vaccine efficacy. On the other hand, one of the most effective ways to decrease transmission is to scale-up vaccination. Within this catch-22 situation, slowing viral transmission and decreasing viral replication is paramount and supersedes concerns about variants. Hence, vaccination in the presence of high transmission is strongly recommended at this time.

4. What does the regular emergence of new COVID-19 variants tell us about the need tovaccinate the global population in order to protect the U.S.?

Although the development of these vaccines provides hope that we can begin to control the spread of SARS-CoV-2, the inequitable distribution and availability of vaccines across the world casts doubt on how rapidly, and even if, some measure of global epidemic control will be achievable. Currently, 77% of all vaccine doses have been administered in just 10 countries (the US, China, India, the UK, Brazil, Turkey, Germany, Indonesia, France and Russia), while some countries are yet to start their SARS-CoV-2 vaccination programs. From a policy and public health perspective, global equitable access to a vaccine, particularly prioritizing protection of healthcare workers and the elderly, is the key to mitigating the worldwide public health and economic impact of the pandemic. Unfortunately, vaccine nationalism has resulted in unequal distribution of and access to SARS-CoV-2 vaccines. The Director-General of the World Health Organization (WHO), Tedros A. Ghebreyesus, has cautioned about this issue, saying "the world is on the brink of a catastrophic moral failure".

The spread of SARS-CoV-2 in one part of the world affects all parts of the world due to extensive global connections. Even for a country with high vaccination rates, if neighboring countries have ongoing high rates of viral transmission as they have not been able to vaccinate so widely or rapidly, new outbreaks could occur and new variants could spread when the populations interact. Defeating the pandemic requires global control, which can only be achieved through the equitable global distribution of vaccines.

In addressing this problem early in the pandemic, the WHO, in collaboration with its partners, launched the Access to Covid-19 Tools (ACT)-Accelerator partnership, which supports efforts to develop tools including diagnostics, treatment, vaccines and health system strengthening to fight Covid-19. The vaccine pillar of the ACT-Accelerator initiative is known as COVAX. Initiated in April 2020 by Gavi, the Coalition for Epidemic Preparedness Innovations (CEPI) and the WHO, COVAX is a global mechanism that invests in the development, manufacturing, procurement and distribution of Covid-19 vaccine candidates, offering member countries equitable access, regardless of income level, to successful vaccines as they become available. At present, the goal of COVAX is to provide countries with enough doses to cover 20% of their populations.

The inequitable distribution of resources significantly undermines the effective management and control of the pandemic. This concern is not hypothetical or theoretical; it was demonstrated by the actions of individual states in the US in March 2020 regarding PPE and ventilators. During that period, the absence of a centralized federal government procurement strategy for these items meant that US states were competing against each other, against the federal government and even against cities to procure the necessary equipment. This resulted in prices being driven up and PPE and ventilators being distributed on the basis of available resources, rather than need, and failure to ensure equitable and effective distribution. Such maldistribution of essential Covid-19 resources leads to the loss of lives.

Exactly the same is true of vaccines. At present there is a limited number of vaccines on the market. As such, supply is fixed, and current models predict that there will only be enough vaccines to cover the world's population by 2023. Countries that can afford to pay higher prices can enter bilateral deals with pharmaceutical companies and negotiate to jump the queue. By doing so, they remove vaccines from the available pool and end up limiting vaccine allocations to other countries, which undermines the objective of systematically vaccinating the highest number of people across the globe in the shortest period of time.

According to the Duke Global Health Innovation Center, to date high-income countries have secured 4.7 billion doses, upper-middle-income countries have secured 1.5 billion doses, lower- middle-income countries have secured 731 million doses and low-income countries have secured 770 million doses. Some low- and middle-income countries (LMICs) with vaccine manufacturing capacity, such as India and Brazil, and those with the infrastructure to host clinical trials, such as Peru, have used those assets as leverage to negotiate purchase deals.

However, most LMICs have not been able to secure enough vaccines.

Pharmaceutical companies, with the exception of J&J, have not adopted a single exit price for their SARS-CoV-2 vaccines. The prices are therefore open to market forces, especially as the use of non-disclosure agreements means that these companies can prevent differential pricing from become public. More demand, especially from countries under significant pressure to buy vaccines, means higher prices. High-income countries with large buying capacity are able to pay higher prices, again pushing lower income countries out of the equation and furthering inequitable distribution.

Vaccine nationalism and the hoarding of vaccines is a consequence of limited supplies. Unfortunately, SARS-CoV-2 vaccines are currently manufactured by just a handful of companies. However, there are vast capabilities throughout the world to manufacture vaccines. For example, in Africa, companies like Biovac and Aspen in South Africa, Institute Pasteur in Senegal and Vacsera in Egypt could rapidly adapt to start making SARS-CoV-2 vaccines if provided with the funding, IP rights and know-how. The reliance of LMICs on others for the development of vaccines as well as diagnostic technologies has also highlighted the dire need for these countries to increase local investments in science and technology to build self- sufficiency and enhance their capacity to control pandemics.

There is a mistaken belief by some countries that they can vaccinate their populations and then they will be safe. This simply is not true. There is no endgame that sees one country achieving sustained control of the virus while the rest of the world is dealing with rampant spread. In the Covid-19 pandemic, no-one is safe until everyone is safe. This pandemic has highlighted the inter-dependence between individuals, between communities and between countries. Each person's risk of infection is influenced as much by the actions of others as it by their own actions. The antidote to vaccine nationalism is the recognition and appreciation of our mutual inter-dependence and the need to act with all our humanity to seek a just and equitable approach to vaccine access to overcome this pandemic.

Annexure 1.

"SARS-CoV-2 variants: the need for urgent public health action beyond vaccines"

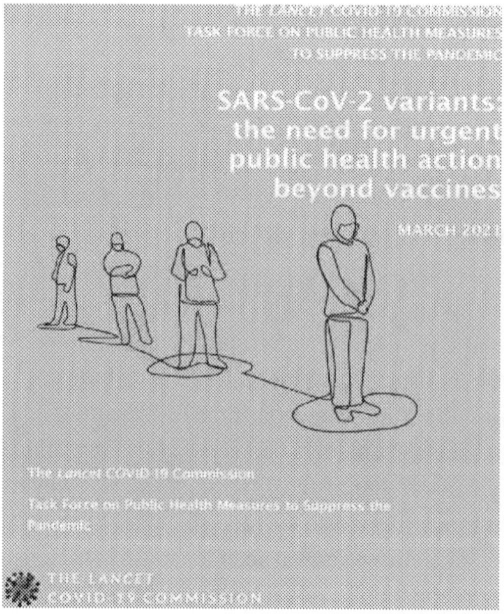

Task Force Members and Staff

Task Force Members

Jong-Koo Lee (Co-chair), Professor, College of Medicine, Seoul National University / Former Director of KCDC, Republic of Korea.

Chris Bullen (Co-chair), Auckland University Population Health, Director of National Institute for Health Innovation, New Zealand.

Salim S. Abdool Karim, Professor of Global Health, Department of Epidemiology, Mailman School of Public Health, Columbia University, South Africa.

Simon Bush, Director of Neglected Tropical Diseases, Sightsavers, Ghana, UK/Ghana.

Francesca Colombo, Head of the Health Division at the OECD, France.

Alejandro Gaviria, President, Universidad de los Andes, Former Minister of Health, Colombia.

John Lavis, Director of the World Health Organisation (WHO) Collaborating Centre for Evidence Informed Policy, Canada.

Jeffrey Lazarus, Professor, Barcelona Institute for Global Health Hospital Clinic - University of Barcelona, Spain.

Yi-Chun Lo, Deputy Director-General, Taiwan Centers for Disease Control, Taiwan.

Susan Michie, Professor, Department of Clinical, Educational and Health Psychology Universtiy College London, UK.

Ole Frithjof Norheim, Professor, Department of Global Public Health and Primary Care University of Bergen, Norway.

Srinath Reddy, Director, Public Health Foundation India, India

María del Rocío Sáenz Madrigal, Professor of health promotion, University of Costa Rica, Former Minister of Health of Costa Rica, Costa Rica.

Mikael Rostila, Professor, Department of Publich Health Science Stockholm University, Sweden.

Liam Smith, Professor, Director of BehaviourWorks Australia, Monash University, Australia.

John Thwaites, Professor, Chair of Monash Sustainable Development Institue Monash University, Australia.

Miriam Khamadi Were, Professor, Vice Chair, The Champions of AIDS-Free Generation, Kenya.

Lan Xue, Distinguished Professor and Dean, Schwarzman College, Tsinghua University, China.

Secretariat and Task Force Staff
Yanis Ben Amor, Assistant Professor of Global Health and Microbiological Sciences, Executive Director, Center for Sustainable Development, Columbia University, USA.
Booyuel Kim, Associate Professor, Graduate School of Environmental Studies, Seoul National University.

Key Points

1. SARS-CoV-2 variants of concern have emergedsimultaneously in many countries, including the highly transmissible variant B.1.351, now present inat least 46 countries.
2. Lack of capacity for genomic surveillance in many countries, including some higher income countries, means that the situation may be even more serious than it appears.
3. No one is safe until everyone is safe. We are in a race against time to get global transmission rateslow enough to prevent the emergence and spread of new variants overcoming immunity conferred by vaccination and prior disease.
4. Differences in the effectiveness of vaccines in providing immunity to variant B.1.351 raises theconcern that current vaccines may be less effectiveagainst new and emerging variants.
5. No single action is sufficient to prevent the spread of the virus: strong public health measures against the virus must be maintained in tandem with global vaccination programs.
6. Conducting clinical trials of vaccines for every highly transmissible variant as it emerges is impracticable given the time needed to conduct them. We urgentlyneed to identify biomarkers that can accurately predict vaccine protection against infection, disease and death.

The Problem

At the end of 2020, there was strong hope that a global vaccination programme would render SARS-CoV-2 an endemic virus that could be contained at very low levels without further societal disruption or significant numbers of deaths. However, SARS-CoV-2 variants of concern have emerged and spread around the world, which means that current pandemic control efforts, including vaccination, are threatened.

Genetic mutations of viruses like SARS-CoV-2 emerge frequently, but some variants are labelled "variants of concern" because they have one or more of the following features:

- They can 're-infect' people who already have antibodies from a previous infection and they can infect people who have already been vaccinated, which has significant potential implications for what current vaccination programs can achieve;
- They are more easily passed from one individual to the next, which has potential implications for public health measures and for health system preparedness (given infections and hospitalizations occur more rapidly); and
- They can lead to more severe disease, which has implications for health system preparedness.
- There are currently at least three documented SARS- CoV-2 variants of concern:
- B.1.351, first reported in South Africa in December 2020;
- B.1.1.7, which was first reported in the U.K. in December 2020;
- P.1, which was first reported in Brazil and Japan.

Experience in South Africa suggests that:

- Past infection with SARS-CoV-2 offers no or only very weak protection against the B.1.351 variants;
- The AstraZeneca vaccine-generated antibodies have up to an 86-fold reduction in neutralizing activity and 3.2-fold lower (70% vs 22%) clinical efficacy against mild to moderate illness for B.1.351; and
- The B.1.351 variant is about 50% more transmissible compared to pre-existing variants.

The B.1.351 variant has already been detected in at least 46 countries, including in the U.S.

If there are high levels of transmission and hence of replication of SARS-CoV-2 anywhere in the world, there will be more variants of concern, with the more infectious variants dominating. With international mobility, these variants will spread. Similar mutations are occurring in different countries simultaneously, meaning that noteven border controls and high vaccination rates can protect individual countries from home-grown variants, including variants of concern, where there is substantial community transmission. Reducing community transmission is therefore paramount.

Need for Urgent Action

1. Maximum suppression: Public health leaders should focus on efforts that maximally suppress viral infection rates and hence preventing the emergence of mutations that can become new variants of concern (each time the virus replicates there is an opportunity for a mutation to occur), through a combination of vaccination and continued public health and behavioural measures (such as facemasks and physical distancing).
2. Global equity in vaccine access: High-income countries should support multilateral mechanisms such as COVAX vaccines and donate excess vaccine to low and middle income countries. They should strengthen laboratory research globally, enable and accelerate knowledge transfer and sharing of intellectual property. While equitable access is an important global goal, there is an overarching imperative to reduce the emergence of viral variants of concern, and this may necessitate prioritising those countries or locations with highest disease prevalence and levels of transmission, where the selective pressure and the rate of mutation are likely to be greatest.
3. Strengthen public health and behavioural interventions: in all countries to reduce the risk of further dangerous variants.
4. Capacity to accommodate surges in demand for healthcare: Health system leaders need to mobilise and support health professionals and manage increased hospitalizations over shorter periods during surges, without reducing care for non-COVID patients.
5. Preparedness: Suppression of viral infection rates and health system efforts need to be accompanied by:
   - Genomic surveillance programmes to identify and quickly characterize emerging variants in as many countries as possible around the world;
   - Rapid large-scale 'second-generation' A vaccine programmes and increased production capacity that can support equity in vaccine distribution across and within countries;
   - Studies of vaccine effectiveness in relation to existing and new variants of concern (ideally using biomarkers in laboratory

studies and rapid clinical studies that yield results quickly) and living syntheses of these studies that derive implications for vaccine choice, combinations and re-vaccination;

- Monitoring of the ability of diagnostic tests to reliably identify new variants;
- Evaluation studies that examine need for adaptation to public health measures (e.g., double masking, duration of quarantine, approach to and frequency of testing) and to health system arrangements (e.g., hospital and long-term care visitor policies, personal protective equipment (PPE), sharing of room or ward by two or more patients who are infected with the same microorganism, Heating Ventilation and Air Conditioning systems, and surge capacity).

***

Chairman FOSTER. Thank you. And next we will recognize Dr. Grubaugh for five minutes.

Statement of Dr. Nathan Grubaugh, Assistant Professor of Epidemiology

Dr. GRUBAUGH. Thank you, Chairman Foster and Members of the Subcommittee, for the invitation to discuss SARS CoV–2 variants. I am a virologist and molecular epidemiologist. That is, I use virus genome sequencing and molecular diagnostic assays to study the emergence and spread of infectious diseases. I helped to develop the SARS-CoV–2 genomic surveillance system for the State of Connecticut and I worked directly with the CDC (Centers for Disease Control and Prevention) and other regional and inter- national partners to investigate the emergence of SARS-CoV–2 variants.

Surveillance is one of our most important tools for public health. Almost all major policy decisions rely on data informing the spread and incidence of an infectious disease. And it's not just local surveillance. We need global surveillance to inform as to what may be coming next. For example, surveillance from South Africa, Brazil, India, and the U.K. have provided critical information about what variants may be introduced into the United

States, which is in addition to the variants that may emerge within our own borders.

While sequencing COVID–19 cases in the United States is increasing, there are still many regions in the world of which we have little or no SARS-CoV–2 genomic information. These gaps lead us into the dark what—as to what variants may be emerging in those locations and what could be a threat to the United States. Local surveillance systems detect variants by the pattern of specific mutation of each sequence virus, which we then use to assigned to a numbered lineage, such is B.1.1.7, B.1.351, P.1, et cetera. These data are then used to detect the introductions and track the fre- quencies of known or novel variants.

Our national and international surveillance systems are then reliant on SARS-CoV–2 genomic sequencing data to be submitted to public repositories. GISAID (Global Initiative on Sharing All Influ- enza Data) is the most popular repository which currently contains about 1.5 million sequences from around the world. From there, bioinformaticists and public health agencies and independent groups routinely poll the data to provide global, national, and regional reports on variants. This allows all of us to keep up-to-date on what is happening.

But there are some major challenges to variant surveillance. One is that it mostly requires the use of whole genome virus sequencing, a method that is far more expensive and technical than conventional clinical testing. There are some simpler tests, similar to what we use for clinical diagnostic testing, that are used to help us to track the frequency of variants. For example, a PCR (polymerase chain reaction) test has been used to track the rapid spread of B.1.1.7 in the United States. These simpler tests, however, are limited in what they can detect. It's hard for them to detect some- thing that is novel. So while useful, they are not a replacement for sequencing.

Another challenge is the need for individual labs to share their data on public repositories. While data sharing is critical to our surveillance efforts, there are several barriers, especially in low-resource settings. These include technical barriers to data transfers to online repositories, lack of important information connected to the sequences needed for public health, lack of incentives to make expensive-to-generate genomic data available to the public versus keeping them for their own research, and international responses to publicly submitted data such as naming a variant after a location or the implementation of travel restrictions.

Here provides an opportunity for the U.S. Government to help. We need policies around pathogen genomic data sharing and usage for public health surveillance. These should include incentives to share and also protections for data generators to have the first right to publish. These policies should also be accompanied by standards for data generation, standards for data processing, and standards for analysis to help minimize sampling biases and eliminate data processing errors.

Finally, these policies should support the work of pathogen genomic surveillance of all types not just during a public health emergency. Without sustained support, the important work that we started here could fold. Rather, our genomic surveillance system should remain intact and only ramp up or ramp down depending on the need.

Thank you for your time, and I hope that I can answer any questions that you may have.

[The prepared statement of Dr. Grubaugh follows:]

Written Statement of Dr. Nathan Grubaugh, Assistant Professor of Epidemiology

Questions presented by the Subcommittee:

1. What is the state of data sharing regarding variants developing and spreading across the globe? How are new variants detected and, once their genomes are sequenced, how is that information proliferated?

SARS-CoV-2 genomes from COVID-19 cases have been sequenced from around the globe since the beginning of pandemic. This process, however, is expensive and technical, and thus there are significant inequities in SARS-CoV-2 genomic data generation. Figure 1 summarizes the percent of COVID-19 cases per week that have been sequenced and shared on a public repository across regions and countries. Australia (AUS), Japan (JPN), Denmark (DNK), and Great Britain (GBR) are some of the only counties that have been able to consistently sequence >5% of the COVID-19 cases, while there is little to no SARS-CoV-2 genomic data from many countries in Asia, Africa, and the Caribbean. The United States has so far sequenced 0.5-1% of the total COVID-19 cases, though sequencing has significantly increased in recent months. These global and national genomic surveillance gaps severely limit our ability to detect new and emerging SARS-CoV-2 variants, and should be considered as a threat to US public health.

SARS-CoV-2 genomic data is primarily shared via GISAID (gisaid.org), and to a lesser extent, other repositories like the National Center for Biotechnology Information (NCBI) Genbank (https://www.ncbi.nlm.nih.gov/sars-cov-2/). As of May 6, 2021, there were 1,432,306 SARS-CoV-2 genome submissions on GISAID, compared to 386,022 on Genbank. It is unclear, however, the percent of the total SARS-CoV-2 genomes that have been sequenced that these databases represent. There are some disincentives for laboratories to not publicly share their SARS-CoV-2 genomic data. This list is not exhaustive, but it includes:

- Technical barriers to data transfers to online repositories.
- Lack of complete metadata (collection date, location, patient information).
- Lack of incentives to make expensive-to-generate genomic data available to the public.
- Lack of protection for the researchers to have first rights to publishing their data.
- Inappropriate international responses to publicly submitted data, such as naming a variant after a location or the implementation of travel restrictions.

Most variants are initially detected by local laboratories or public health agencies. The SARS-CoV-2 genomic data are processed through open software like Pangolin (https://pangolin.cog-uk.io/) or Nextclade (https://clades.nextstrain.org/) that assign each sequenced to a specific lineage or clade based on the specific mutations in each sequence. This provides an output such as "B.1.1.7" and a list of mutations. Many local laboratories or public health agencies are consistently monitoring the lineage assignments to (1) detect novel lineages that contain one or more mutations of interest, (2) detect the outside introduction of a known variant of concern or interest, and (3) track the frequencies of locally circulating variants.

There are also efforts to monitor for variants on national and global scales. There are now several programs, such as Outbreak.info (https://outbreak.info/situation-reports) and Nextstrain (https://nextstrain.org/) that pull data from GISAID daily to allow the user to generate custom variant tracking reports. Routine GISAID data retrievals are also used for many state and national surveillance programs to provide updates on the number of specific variants of concern or interest (e.g., https://covid.cdc.gov/covid-data-tracker/#variant-proportions). The outputs of these reports are presented on various platforms, including press releases, traditional media, and social media.

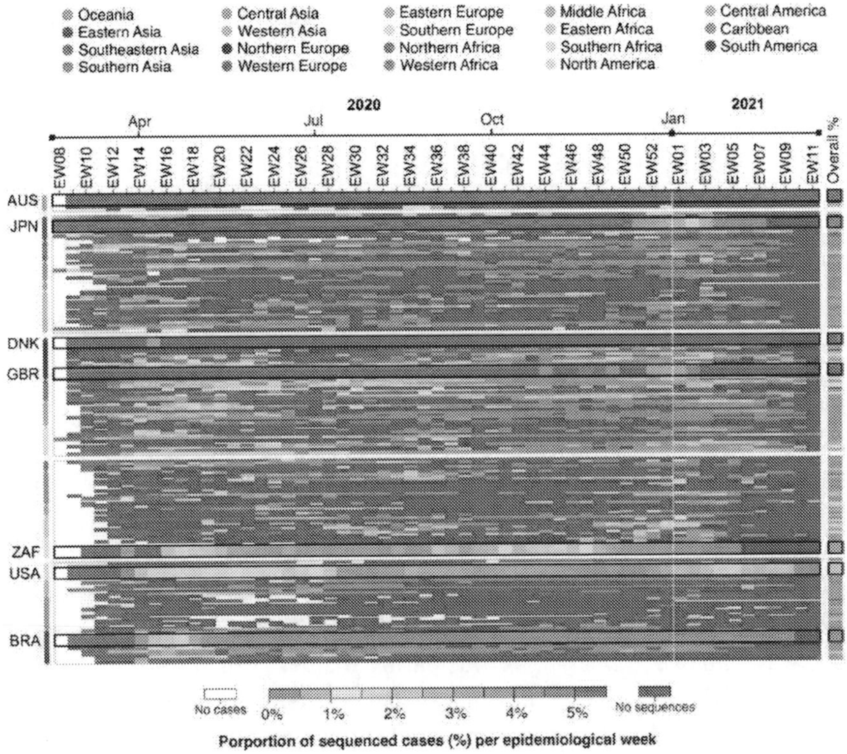

Figure 1. Proportion of sequenced cases per country per epidemiological week, 2020-2021 (up to April 16th, 2021). Few countries have capacity to sequence more than 5% of reported cases with genome coverage >/= 70%, especially when COVID-19 incidence is high. When incidence is low, as in early phases of the pandemic, most countries were able to sequence high proportions of cases (3-5%, green and blue shades). However, with the aggravation of the pandemic, few countries were able to keep up, and in poor countries, despite cases being reported, many weeks had few (red) or no sequences (grey).
Figure created by Anderson Brito, PhD (postdoctoral associate in the Grubaugh Laboratory at the Yale School of Public Health).

2. Are existing COVID-19 tests effective at diagnosing infections of known variants? How are variant-specific tests use to bolster public health decision-making?

To my knowledge, all known SARS-CoV-2 variants can still be detected by the common clinical diagnostic assays. While some deletions or mutations can impact individual diagnostic assay targets, most clinical diagnostic assays target multiple parts of the genome to overcome this issue. Thus there is not currently a significant issue with variants causing inconclusive or false negative results. However, this is an area to continuously monitor, and there are several ongoing and parallel efforts to track mutations in diagnostic targets.

The primary issue is that standard diagnostics cannot differentiate between SARS-CoV-2 variants. While whole genome sequencing is the gold standard for variant identification, the additional time, expense, and laboratory equipment make sequencing not practical in all circumstances. PCR and other less complicated assays have the ability to detect a limited number of virus mutations, which can be indicative of a limited set of variants. These assays, which can be faster, cheaper, and less complicated, have an advantage of being able to generate information about variant frequencies with shorter turnaround times and at a larger scale than whole genome sequencing.

For example, the SARS-CoV-2 variant B.1.1.7 has a 6 nucleotide deletion in its spike protein, which causes a spike gene target failure (SGTF) result in one of the three targets with the ThermoFisher TaqPath COVID-19 Combo Kit. The result is still valid, but by comparing the number of positive results with and without SGTF, we can get a relative picture of B.1.1.7 prevalence. This was valuable in tracking the increasing frequency of B.1.1.7 in the UK, and it is now being used in the US. National data about B.1.1.7 provenance based on TaqPath SGTF results are provided by Helix. My group also uses SGTF results to help track the frequency of B.1.1.7 in Connecticut (Figure 2; https://covidtrackerct.com/variant-surveillance/).

PCR assays specific to other variants have been developed, which can provide similar results to the above for B.1.1.7. These assays can be the most beneficial when they are used as the primary diagnostic test to immediately provide a SARS-CoV-2 test result and some information about the variant, rather than an add-on test. Variant-specific assays, however, cannot detect novel variants, and thus should only compliment whole genome sequencing, and not replace.

3. How can the federal government serve as a resource during and between pandemics when it comes to information aggregation and accessibility?

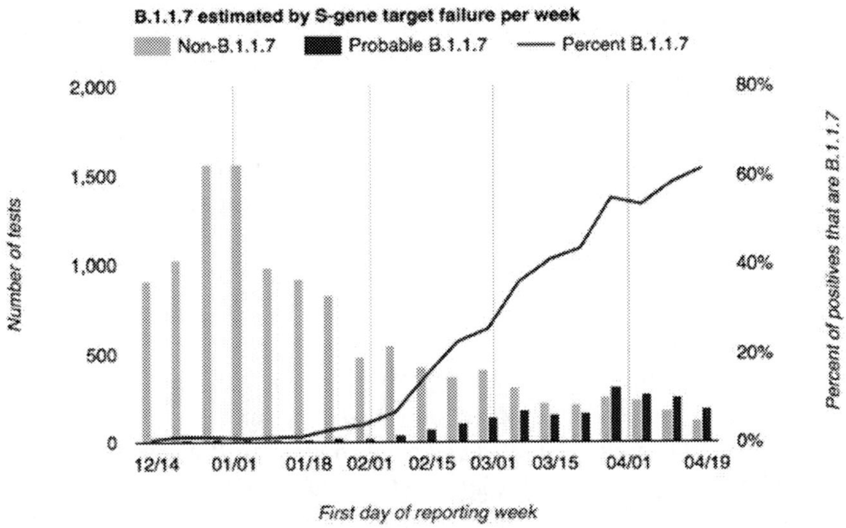

Figure 2. Presumed B.1.1.7 positivity (%). Tests performed by Yale-New Haven Hospital (primary catchment = NewHaven and Fairfield Counties, CT) and Jackson Labs (primary catchment = New Haven and Hartford Counties, CT).
Probable B.1.1.7 positivity defined as "spike gene target failure" (SGTF) frequency on the TaqPath SARS-CoV-2 diagnostic test. Figure from Covid Tracker CT (https://covidtrackerct.com/variant-surveillance/).

In my opinion, there are three primary ways that the federal government can facilitate data aggregation and accessibility during pandemics: policy, standards, and support.

The first is policy based. In my response to question 1, I outlined some barriers to pathogen data being shared on public repositories. It is not mandatory for data generated during pandemics that can benefit public health to be shared publicly. Furthermore, there are no policies in place to protect the rights of the data generators to have the first rights to publish the data. My group openly shares the genomic data that we generate in hopes that public health agencies can use it for decision making but also in hope that other academic labs will not scoop our data in their publication. Because some data (like sequencing data) can be very expensive to generate and publications are the "currency" for academic advancement, many groups are not open to sharing their data out of self preservation. Thus we often find data released upon a paper's acceptance in a journal. While data sharing during the COVID-19 pandemic has been exceptional, these problems continue to exist. Thus finding resolutions around the legality of data sharing and usage to create an equitable framework would enhance data sharing during future pandemics.

Second, many forms of data useful for public health, including pathogen genomic sequencing, can be generated, processed, and analyzed by applying a variety of controls and methods. Then compiling data generated among different laboratories can create biases and inaccurate findings because they may represent different populations, include different intrinsic errors, or have different definitions/classifications of data fields. Thus standardization is critical, and is only likely to come from the national level. The federal government could create panels of field-specific experts to provide standards for sample selection, data generation, computational processing, and associated metadata.

Most importantly, public health surveillance - including all aspects from data collection, generation, storage, and dissemination - needs to be fully supported outside of outbreak/epidemic/pandemic times. We have seen many "pop-up" efforts created to fill critical needs, and some of this can be alleviated with consistent support. For example, many of the online tools mentioned above (e.g., outbreak.info) were created to assist with the pandemic response, and some of them may not be supported for long after the pandemic. If the national agencies can learn from the openness and innovation of the private and academic initiatives, they may be able to help preserve these tools and expand their use beyond SARS-CoV-2. As another example, the generation of and consistent support for NCBI means that there is a database to obtain access to records and data, which is fundamental for research and public health. Expanding these programs to include surveillance data which is notoriously difficult to obtain would help to ensure that we have systems in place for when there are public healthemergencies.

Dr. Nathan Grubaugh is Assistant Professor of Epidemiology at the Yale School of Public Health and head of the Grubaugh Lab studying virus emergence, transmission, and evolution. His lab uses genomics to determine the emergence risk and to track the spread of mosquito-borne viruses. Specifically, the lab sequences viruses during outbreaks for epidemiological investigations (genomic epidemiology), determines the disease phenotype and transmission fitness of novel virus mutations that occur during outbreaks (functional genomics), and maps the evolutionary pathways that a virus may take to adapt to a new environment (experimentalevolution). Their goals are to integrate genomic data into surveillance and response programs to better prevent and control future mosquito-borne virus outbreaks.

Dr. Grubaugh earned his PhD in microbiology with a focus on West Nile virus evolution from Colorado State University in 2016 and went on to be a postdoctoral fellow at The Scripps Research Institute to study the 2015-2017

Zika virus epidemic. He also has a MS in biotechnology from Johns Hopkins University. Prior to graduate school, he spent around 7 yearsworking in the biotech industry doing toxicology studies, monitoring food production lines for pathogens, and developing early phase vaccine candidates.

***

Chairman FOSTER. Thank you. And the Chair will now recognize Dr. Streiffer for five minutes.

Statement of Dr. Stephen Streiffer, Deputy Laboratory Director for Science and Technology, Argonne National Laboratory

Dr. STREIFFER. Chairwoman Johnson, Chairman Foster, Ranking Member Obernolte, Members of the Subcommittee, thank you for the opportunity to testify today about the challenges presented by the COVID–19 variants and the important role the Department of Energy's national laboratories have played in combating COVID– 19.

My name is Dr.—as Congressman Foster said, I'm Stephen Streiffer. I serve as Argonne's—National Laboratory's Deputy Laboratory Director for Science and Technology, as well as the Director of the lab's Advanced Photon Source (APS). For the last 15 months it's been my privilege to serve as the Co-Director of the DOE's National Virtual Biotechnology Laboratory.

As, again, Congressman Foster pointed out, the NVBL came together as a consortium of all 17 DOE national laboratories at the onset of the pandemic, supported by *CARES Act* funding. It brought together leading scientists and researchers from across the lab complex and leverages the Department of Energy's world-class experimental and computational facilities. Our state-of-the-art user facilities such as the APS, our capabilities in advanced computing and AI (artificial intelligence), structural and molecular biology and biotechnology, epidemiological and transportation modeling and advanced manufacturing, among others, uniquely position us to take on this challenge and lead the world in finding therapies to combat the virus.

If you'll allow me, I'll just go through several of the contributions that NVBL has made in the fight against COVID. I'll highlight just a few here, and there's more in my written testimony of course.

As the Nation initially grappled with testing, the lab supported the FDA, CDC, and DOD (Department of Defense) to establish national guidelines, identify diagnostic targets, and develop and prove out sample collection methodologies that were used in the administration of hundreds of millions of COVID–19 tests. We also worked to solve supply chain challenges that plagued the early days of the outbreak. Teams from the NVBL produced innovations in materials and advanced manufacturing that mitigated shortages and test kit components and personal protective equipment, leading to the creation of over 1,000 new jobs as we transferred development to the private sector. Our high-performance computing and AI capabilities have proven extremely effective in the molecular design of medical therapeutics and in epidemiological mobility modeling to support decisionmakers.

As far as we've come in the fight against COVID–19, as we're here today to discuss, the biggest threat right now are the variants that are emerging around the globe. An integrated approach that tracks and responds to the variants is what we need at this stage of the pandemic.

Written Statement of Dr. Stephen Streiffer, Deputy Laboratory Director for Science and Technology, Argonne National Laboratory

Chairman Foster, Ranking Member Obernolte, and Members of the Subcommittee, thank you for the invitation to testify before you today about the critical role of the U.S. Department of Energy (DOE) national laboratories in combatting the COVID-19 pandemic and the virus' emerging variants. My name is Stephen Streiffer and I serve as Argonne National Laboratory's deputy laboratory director for science and technology, as well as the director of the lab's Advanced Photon Source.

For the last 15 months I have also had the honor of serving as the co-director of the DOE's National Virtual Biotechnology Laboratory (NVBL). The NVBL is truly one of the unsung heroes in the nation's fight against this disease. It was formed at the beginning of the pandemic to put the broad capabilities of the DOE complex to the task of fighting COVID-19, including the expertise and facilities of all 17 DOE national laboratories. Our labs are home to scientists and researchers that lead the world in their areas of expertise. We also house unique and powerful "user facilities": experimental and computational tools used by researchers from universities, government laboratories, and companies from across the country and around the world.

The national laboratories have a long history of putting our groundbreaking discoveries and innovations to work responding to national and international emergencies. From the 2005 Hurricane Katrina disaster, to the 2010 Deepwater Horizon oil spill, to the 2011 Fukushima nuclear accident, we have been on the front lines, helping with immediate response and developing long-term technical solutions. When the COVID-19 pandemic hit, we were prepared, ready, and willing to support an whole-of-government effort to fight the disease.

Accomplishments of the NVBL in Fighting COVID-19

The creation of the NVBL allowed the laboratories' collective capabilities to be almost immediately transformed into key assets in the world's fight against COVID-19. With funding from the CARES Act, all 17 national laboratories, through the NVBL, addressed medical supply shortages, discovered potential drugs to fight the virus, developed and verified COVID-19 testing methods, modeled disease spread and impact locally and nationally, and helped officials understand virus transport in buildings and the environment. Although NVBL CARES Act funding has been fully expended, this work sets the stage for ongoing work to identify, understand, track, and treat variants.

The national laboratory resources leveraged for this effort include a suite of world-leading facilities that are used by scientists from universities, industry, and other laboratories across the country and around the world:

- Light and neutron sources
- Nanoscale science research centers
- Sequencing and biocharacterization facilities
- High-performance computing centers
- Advanced manufacturing research facilities

Here are a few of the many contributions that the NVBL has made to the fight against COVID-19, through both the labs' discoveries and innovations and the support of their user facilities to the international scientific community.

Molecular Design for Medical Therapeutics

DOE's high-performance computers and light and neutron sources were used to identify promising candidates for antibodies and antivirals that universities and drug companies are now evaluating. These efforts were led by Oak Ridge, Lawrence Berkeley, and Lawrence Livermore National Laboratories with participation from six other laboratories. Specific examples include:

- Used artificial intelligence methods to screen 1040 (over a thousand-trillion-trillion-trillion) possible antibody variations, identifying the best matches against the SARS-CoV-2 spike protein.
- Computationally screened tens of millions of small molecules against SARS-CoV-2 viral proteins and then experimentally evaluated top contenders, greatly accelerating the search for new antiviral therapeutics.

Development and Evaluation of COVID-19 Testing

NVBL researchers developed new diagnostic targets and sample collection approaches and supported U.S. Food and Drug Administration (FDA), Centers for Disease Control and Prevention (CDC), and Department of Defense (DoD) efforts to establish national guidelines used in administering hundreds of millions of COVID-19 tests. Led by Los Alamos, Sandia, and Lawrence Livermore National Laboratories, with significant contributions from eight other laboratories, projects included:

- Collaborated with DoD, CDC, and FDA to provide experimental data in support of national testing guidelines, assessing potential contamination in commercial kits, evaluating protocols such as for pooled samples, examining test kit viral transport media and protocols, and evaluating virus inactivation and extraction methods. These projects helped ensure that the nation was using effective tests and protocols and protecting frontline health care workers.
- Developed tools to analyze and assess how variants of the SARS-CoV-2 virus may affect the reliability of COVID-19 tests.

Epidemiological and Transportation Modeling

Researchers used artificial intelligence and high-performance computing to produce near real-time analysis of data to forecast disease transmission, stress on public health infrastructure, and impacts to the economy and transportation networks, supporting decision-makers at the local, state, and national levels. This work informed pandemic response with respect to underserved communities in Illinois, New Mexico, and Tennessee. Led by Oak Ridge National Laboratory with participation from six other laboratories (Argonne, Lawrence Berkeley, Livermore, Los Alamos, National Renewable Energy Laboratory, and Sandia), specific projects include:

- Created an approach to forecast COVID-19 case counts at state, county, and metropolitan scalesusing data-driven statistical models, enabling short-term planning of contact tracing, healthcarestaffing, testing capacity, and vaccination strategies.
- Performed longer-term, scenario-based analysis and mitigation planning to support decisionmakers with information on effects of nonmedical interventions such as social distancing, masking, stay-at-home policies, and school closures before they are implemented.
- Collected and curated disease data, which created a unique national data resource to support epidemiological and pandemic modeling, including assessment of the impact of human behavioron infection spread and location and the availability of critical infrastructure.
- Developed an approach using cellular phone- and vehicle-derived data to reveal transportation patterns across industries, including bars and restaurants, as well as passenger, fleet, and heavy-duty vehicles.

Viral Fate and Transport

NVBL teams studied how to control indoor virus movement to minimize uptake and protect human health, designed materials to deactivate the virus, and developed models to track it in wastewater. This effort was led by Pacific Northwest National Laboratory with strong participation from Lawrence Berkeley, Livermore, and eight other laboratories. Examples include:

- Provided critical information about how behavioral, environmental, and operational conditions affect the risk of airborne virus transmission indoors, such as in classrooms, offices, and conference rooms, to mitigate viral spread in enclosed spaces.
- Designed new antiviral materials that can deactivate the virus.
- Produced and validated models for SARS-CoV-2 fate and transport in wastewater, enabling wastewater sampling as a means to provide

early warning and hot-spot detection of localized COVID-19 outbreaks.

Advanced Manufacturing

Within just a few months, NVBL teams produced innovations in materials and advanced manufacturing that mitigated shortages in test kit components and personal protective equipment (PPE), creating over 1,000 new jobs. All 17 national laboratories contributed, and specific partnerships with industry include:

- Designed a system for mass producing N95 filter media, enabling Cummins Filtration (Nashville, TN) to produce material for more than 3 million masks per day, and worked with DemeTech (Miami Lakes, FL) to convert the N95 material to masks and respirators.
- Worked with the U.S. Department of Health and Human Services and Coca-Cola (Atlanta, GA), which produces 2 billion bottle preforms per week, to evaluate the use of these preforms to alleviate shortages of test tubes used to collect nasal swab samples.
- Developed an approach to 3D print the tooling needed to produce over 8 million sample collection tubes weekly by Thermo Fisher Scientific, Inc. (Lenexa, KS).
- Developed a new low-cost ventilator with BioMedInnovations (Denver, NC) that received FDA Emergency Use Authorization approval.

These accomplishments, made possible through the NVBL, demonstrate the game-changing resource represented by DOE's 17 national laboratories working together virtually, with a single focus on alleviating pandemic challenges. Going forward, the NVBL can bring these resources to bear on future national and international needs and emergencies.

Basic Research Underlies COVID-19 Vaccines

The speed with which effective COVID-19 vaccines were developed and disseminated has been unprecedented—and it wouldn't have happened without decades of investment in scientific research involving the national laboratories. I share the following two examples.

First, the science behind the production of messenger RNA, or mRNA, that is used in the Pfizer/BioNTech and Moderna vaccines, is based on the building blocks of innovation that started at Brookhaven National Laboratory in the 1980s. At that time, a team led by F. William Studier was studying a virus that attacks E. coli bacteria. They created the first complete sequence of that virus' genome, which allowed them to understand how it produced many copies of itself. Studier and his team learned how to direct this copying capability toward making other things: specifically, copious amounts of RNA. This RNA could be delivered to the ribosomes in cells to be translated into proteins—or used directly in mRNA-based vaccines. Thus, Studier's pivotal discovery almost four decades ago enabled the production of today's life-saving treatments.

Second, five of the vaccines now in use—including those developed by Pfizer/BioNTech, Moderna, and Johnson & Johnson—leverage a technique developed from more than a decade of research at Argonne's Advanced Photon Source (APS). This technique, which increases the effectiveness of the vaccines, was developed by researchers now at the University of Texas at Austin and the National Institute of Allergy and Infectious Diseases, part of the National Institutes of Health (NIH). Their current work on COVID-19 vaccines is based on their research into an entirely different disease: respiratory syncytial virus (RSV), which affects thousands of individuals per year. In their work to develop a vaccine for RSV, they used data from the APS to design a version of an RSV viral protein that would provide an effective target for the immune system, helping it build immunity against the virus. They realized that the technique could be applied to coronaviruses as well, and in 2013 began work on a vaccine for the Middle East Respiratory Syndrome coronavirus (MERS-CoV). They reported success in 2017, which again was supported by their use of the APS. When SARS-CoV-2 emerged, they joined with other researchers to successfully apply the same technique to vaccines against it.

COVID-19 Variants: Strategy and Challenges

Having made great strides in combatting the original SARS-CoV-2 virus, the U.S. and the world is in the midst of a race between human ingenuity and the evolving coronavirus. The growing number of vaccines that have received the FDA's Emergency Use Authorization offer real hope for increasing rates of immunity. However, community prevalence of COVID-19 conversely enables the rise of new virus variants, such as the B.1.1.7 variant first identified in the UK or the B.1.351 variant first identified in South Africa. The DOE national laboratories can build on previously mentioned contributions and continue to drive innovation and information for the sustained, multi-pronged approach necessary to stay ahead in the race against coronavirus mutation.

The SARS-CoV-2 virus, as with any biological entity, is essentially a moving target. As the virus replicates within its host, it will frequently make mistakes – spelling errors – as it copies its genetic code, creating new variants. Many of these mistakes are inconsequential, akin to spelling differences between

American English and British English (e.g., "color" versus "colour"). You can still understand the underlying meaning of the word. Most mutations are benign, although occasionally a spelling mistake is made that is more profound (e.g., "fowl" to "foul"). Thus, some mutations can compound and create a situation where not only has the word's meaning changed but that of the entire sentence as well. At this stage, the virus might not be "readable" by diagnostic tests, and, in the worst case scenario, the vaccine target and therapeutic target might no longer be recognizable.

Protecting our communities from COVID-19 variants can be summarized in four steps. Each of these steps is a complex, research- and technology-intensive process that requires a whole-of-government approach to succeed.

1. Sequence the genome of the virus collected from as many samples as possible, with testingdistributed equally across the country.
2. Provide a centralized inventory of collected viral sequences and build a "family tree" that represents how they relate to each other. This large-scale analysis enables us to understandwhat variants are arising, where they are arising, and when they are arising.
3. Use computational modeling and experimental assessments to identify which variants may escape detection through currently available tests, can evade current vaccines, may be moredangerous, or resist current medical therapeutics.
4. Design new tests, vaccines, and treatments that target and work against variants as theycontinue to emerge.

Through the NVBL, DOE national laboratories are leveraging their resources to provide solutions to all four of these critical steps.

Sequencing and Monitoring Viral Variants

What helps us monitor and identify variants that evade vaccines and therapies is to sequence as many samples of the virus as we can from as many communities as possible, either from testing or from wastewater – in a broad and consistent effort – that allows us to effectively track these changes. We canmake our specialized scientific facilities available to our partners at the NIH, CDC and other agencies to improve and speed up current virus sequencing. We also have expertise in large-scale sampling that can be put to work to support testing across the country.

Analyzing the Virus' "Family Tree"

A framework for comparing, classifying, and analyzing the genome sequences of all of these variants is crucial. This framework is already in place by using phylogenetic trees ("family trees") to represent how the variants are related to one another. Each leaf on the tree represents a variant. Leaves attached to the same twig are very similar, whereas leaves on different branches are less similar. Having this framework in place allows us to understand how certain variants arise and what series of mutations create the path to a certain outcome, such as increased virulence. Although this analogy appears quite simple, the underlying calculations for representing these relationships when considering all of the leaves in the tree is extremely complex. DOE supercomputing resources have historically been a critical component for this type of large-scale bioinformatic analytical work, and they will continue to support this work moving forward. An NIH-funded Bioinformatics Resource Center supported by supercomputing at Argonne provides an ongoing analysis of all emerging variants based on available SARS-CoV-2 genome sequences. As these sequences become available, specific variants of concern are tracked, as are the corresponding discrete changes in their genome sequence that differentiate them.

Identifying Variants of Concern

The DOE national laboratories also play a major role in identifying variants that may escape detection or be resistant to vaccines or treatment. Having the above framework in place in order to identify, classify, and track variants of SARS-CoV-2 also means that this information can be used to understand the implications of these changes on the human body.

We have unique, large-scale scientific facilities – such as the aforementioned light sources – and the corresponding expertise for structural biology work that can identify the actual physical changes in the shape of variant components. If the virus is considered as a set of LEGO bricks, we have the tools to literally manufacture and then inspect each individual brick at the scale of its individual atoms. These bricks are viral proteins. Any change in shape of one of those bricks means that we can predict how it interacts with other bricks, including those that stick to surfaces of human cells. Visualizing the changes in shapes of viral proteins provides insight into how they interact with and function in the human body.

Once we can predict how the changed viral proteins interact in the body, our large-scale computing and data management facilities can quickly assess if existing tests, vaccines, and therapeutics might fail against a new variant.

Mitigating Impacts of New Variants

For the fourth step, designing new testing, protocols, and treatment, the DOE laboratories collectively bring significant resources and expertise to the table. We support computational modeling, data analysis, and artificial intelligence techniques that accelerate the discovery of drugs that can successfully treat COVID variants. Our structural and experimental biology expertise and facilities can help national laboratory and university researchers refine or, if necessary, completely redesign therapeutic antibodies and small molecules in response to variations in the virus.

We can develop new tests for rapid detection of variants in clinical and environmental samples. We can also help decision-makers understand how the virus is transported, so that physical and administrative protocols can be developed and implemented that protect people against variants.

We can provide epidemiological modeling for near real-time forecasts and predictions. These forecasts help officials at all levels plan for different intervention options to prevent COVID variants from spreading, allowing them to make the best decisions regarding how to use their resources to keep our communities healthy. At Argonne, we have supported elected officials from the City of Chicago and the State of Illinois with forecasts and predictions since the start of the COVID pandemic, and stand ready to continue this support for COVID variants.

Lastly, to support both the ongoing response to the pandemic caused by the original SARS-CoV-2 virus, and the new variants, we will continue to develop innovative materials and manufacturing processes that address critical supply chain issues and support domestic production of key supplies.

Challenges and Hurdles

We have come a long way in the last year but we still have far to go both in confronting the current pandemic and preparing the nation for the next one. DOE and the NVBL can play a leading role addressing key concerns including virus sequencing, vaccine hesitancy, speed of drug design, testing and diagnostic development, enhancing epidemiology models, and real-time data sharing.

1. *Virus sequencing.* The U.S. has not performed much in the way of systematic sequencing of the virus in the country's population to identify and track the emergence of variants, and what we have conducted has predominately been done on a regional basis. A national, uniform sequencing of the virus across the whole country is needed to track these emerging variants. Fortunately, the NIH is putting resources into this effort, but more is needed.
2. *Vaccine hesitancy.* Improved public education about the efficacy of vaccines and the pivotal rolethey play in curtailing the extent and length of the pandemic would go a long way towards instilling confidence among the American people and decrease their skepticism about taking thevaccine. The DOE plays an important role in building scientific literacy among the American public, and the laboratories are actively engaged in STEM outreach across communities, including the most underserved. In addition, vaccine uptake/hesitancy is one variable the labs' epidemiological models can address, helping government and public health leaders better understand the likely evolution of the pandemic.
3. *Computational modeling and drug design.* The national laboratories' computational and artificial intelligence tools can accelerate the process of drug and vaccine development, and narrow the field of effective existing treatments. NVBL sponsored projects built computational discovery platforms that leveraged investments from multiple agencies and had demonstrable success in finding potential therapeutics that can enable faster response to future variations.
4. *Testing and diagnostic tool development.* DOE has the capabilities to further evaluate and validate existing or experimental tools for testing and diagnostics. DOE has a long history of experience in large-scale sampling and DNA sequencing and can deploy efforts to lower the costand introduce simpler diagnostics.

5. *Continued epidemiology work.* Artificial intelligence inspired new ways of thinking about data inputs into pandemic models, including data on mobility, health, behavior, and demographics. Future work can incorporate the emergence of vaccine-resistant variants, the analysis of societalimpacts, the effects of international travel, and the potential benefits of vaccination to inform long-term planning efforts to mitigate effects of COVID-19.
6. *Standards and data sharing.* Metropolitan and state-level models of COVID-19 variant-penetration, immunity, transmission, and morbidity/mortality—broken down by geography and demographics—will continue to enhance the nation's ability to proactively plan and near realtime respond to the evolving landscape. These efforts would build on multiple agency investments for a dynamic, accurate, and multi-modal operational picture and provide web- based tools and actionable information for a whole of government approach.

Conclusion

For these reasons, Congress should consider continuing to strongly support the DOE complex and the NVBL as part of the nation's continued response to COVID-19 and future pandemics. At the national laboratories, we have infrastructure, networks, and teams of experts ready to deploy. Together, our national labs were able to develop vaccines, mitigation strategies, and solutions in record time due to Congress's robust and consistent support for the past several decades. Our all-hands approach— marshalling the talent and resources of the national laboratories, other government agencies, pharmaceutical industries, and universities from across the country—was instrumental to the impact we've demonstrated.

We were fortunate that we had a head start on research and modeling of coronaviruses. We were able to develop potential vaccines within weeks of the release of the original virus genomic code (most of the time to the authorization of the vaccines was taken up by Phase 1, 2, and 3 clinical testing). This will not always be the case. In the future, we may be confronted with more complex, less understood, more deadly viruses—diseases that can spread from different species and more effectively evade current treatments.

I am proud of the accomplishments of the NVBL and the national laboratories in responding to the COVID-19 pandemic, and feel confident these resources will be available to respond to future national challenges.

At Argonne, as we celebrate our 75th year as a national lab, we look forward to confronting the next 75 years of complex challenges facing society like the current pandemic. The scale of our facilities, the depth of our experience, and our collaborative approach, which are hallmarks of our national laboratories, match the scale of the pandemic we collectively face, and whatever the future holds.

Thank you to the Subcommittee for your time and consideration. I am happy to answer any questions.

***

Chairman FOSTER. Thank you. And we will now recognize Dr. Rivers for five minutes.

Statement of Dr. Caitlin Rivers, Senior Scholar, Johns Hopkins Center for Health Security

Dr. RIVERS. Chairman Foster, Ranking Member Obernolte, Chairwoman Johnson, and Members of the Subcommittee, thank you for the opportunity to speak to you today about variants and evolving research needs.

In the United States we have entered a new phase of the pandemic. Nearly 60 percent of American adults have begun vaccination, including more than 80 percent of adults over age 65. However, in the last 14 months, over 575,000 Americans have died and 32 million cases have been reported. Beyond the direct impacts, we've endured severe economic consequences, disruption to education, and strain on our healthcare systems. We've collectively suffered an enormous loss, and that grief will not be easily overcome. The situation in some other countries is much worse, and the pandemic is far from over. Case counts globally are reaching new highs. India is in the midst of a terrible wave and reports suggest that in some communities the situation is dire. A variant of interest, B.1.617, may be contributing to the surge. As our own domestic outlook improves, we must turn our attention to helping the world. And as we continue the work of ending the pandemic both at home and abroad, we must also identify the changes necessary to ensure we are never caught in this position again. In doing so, we should recognize that we were caught unprepared more than once. We were unprepared to manage the emergence and swift global spread of the novel coronavirus, and we were late to recognize when it reached our shores. Those delays set us on a worse trajectory than we might have otherwise faced.

But so, too, were we unprepared for variants. Although genomics experts had warned of the threat, it was not until the United Kingdom suffered a severe wave attributed to the B.1.1.7 variant that public health officials worldwide sharpened their focus. B.1.1.7 is now understood to be perhaps 50 percent more transmissible than other variants, and it may also cause more severe illness. The U.K. was able to identify and track this variant over time because they invested heavily in genomic surveillance. That capability yielded important information they needed to guide their response, and they provided warning to the world about what was to come. We did not have that level of genomic surveillance in the United States, and that was a gap.

The United States currently recognizes five variants of concern and several variants of interest. The most concerning possibility with some of these variants is that they may exhibit some degree of immune escape, meaning that vaccines and therapeutics may be somewhat less effective. Future variants may drift even further from the protection existing vaccines can provide, cause more severe illness, or impact diagnostic testing. If we do need to update our vaccines or diagnostics to be a better match, we must know that as early as possible so that we can begin the work—that work before the variant becomes widespread. We must not again be caught unprepared.

The American Rescue Plan includes $1.7 billion for genomic surveillance, as well as additional funds for biological research, expansion of the public health workforce, and a suite of other important public health initiatives that will improve our preparedness, including for variants. Looking ahead, given that SARS CoV–2 is likely to continue to circulate and in anticipation of the next viral threat that we will almost certainly face, Congress should provide long-term, sustainable support for this expansion in our public health infrastructure so that we will be in a better position to respond next time.

As we advance our genomic surveillance infrastructure, we should also further develop the modeling and analytics infrastructure that will allow us to make even better use of that data. With the exception of a few small groups within the Department of Health and Human Services, most modelers work in academia and volunteer to support the public health response when an urgent need arises. This arrangement is not well-suited to either party. The Federal Government would benefit from a permanent capability with infectious disease modelers working to advance the state of the science and support public health decisionmaking both between and during emergencies.

The Biden Administration announced a National Security Directive 1, an intention to create a National Center for Epidemic Forecasting and Outbreak Analytics, and the American Rescue Plan appropriated $500 million to CDC for disease forecasting and data modernization. These are promising steps toward modernizing our response capabilities, and I believe they will serve the Nation well. Congress could help by appropriating annual funding and authorizing language so that the forecasting center can endure as a permanent capability.

In conclusion, although the currently circulating variants complicated our course through the spring months, we are now on track to regain control of the pandemic in the United States. Continued vigilance to current and future variants is essential to ensuring that we maintain our current encouraging trajectory. We must expand our genomic surveillance efforts domestically and work with partners and allies abroad to ensure global coverage. The United States is a world leader in science and technology, and we have the opportunity using those capabilities to lead the world through the rest of the pandemic. Thank you.

[The prepared statement of Dr. Rivers follows:]

Written Statement of Dr. Caitlin Rivers, Senior Scholar, Johns Hopkins Center for Health Security

Current Situation

In the United States, we have entered a new phase of the pandemic. Nearly 60% of American adults have begun vaccination, including more than 80% of adults over age 65. Community transmission is declining, and I believe that by summer we will be able to resume most normal activities. However, in the last 14 months over 575,000 Americans have died and 32 million cases have been reported, with more likely unrecognized. Beyond the direct impacts, we have also endured severe economic consequences, disruption to education, strain on our healthcare systems, and we have missed time with loved ones. We have collectively suffered an enormous loss, and that grief will not be easily overcome. The toll of this pandemic is profound.

The situation in some other countries is much worse, and the pandemic is far from over. Case counts are reaching new highs, with some recent days exceeding 800,000 reported cases and 13,000 deaths. India is in the midst of a terrible wave, and reports suggest that in some communities the situation is dire. A variant of interest, B.1.617, may be contributing to the surge. As our own domestic outbreak improves, we must turn our attention to helping the world.

As we continue the work of ending the pandemic both at home and around the world, we must also identify the changes necessary to ensure we are never in this position again. In doing so, we should recognize that we were caught unprepared more than once. We were unprepared to manage the emergence and swift global spread of the novel coronavirus, and we were late to recognize when it reached our shores. Those delays set us on a worse trajectory than we might have otherwise faced. Strengthening those early-response capabilities will likely feature heavily in reforms.

But so, too, were we unprepared for variants. Although genomics experts had warned of the threat, it was not until the United Kingdom suffered a severe wave attributed to the B.1.1.7 variant that public health officials worldwide sharpened their focus. B.1.1.7 is now understood to be perhaps 50% more transmissible than other variants, and it may also cause more severe illness. The UK was able to identify and track this variant over time because they invested heavily in genomic surveillance, aiming to sequence 10% of their positive cases. That capability yielded important information needed to guide their domestic response. It also provided warning to the world about what was to come. We did not have that level of genomic surveillance in the United States, and that is a gap.

As anticipated, B.1.1.7 has gone on to become dominant in the United States, constituting perhaps 60% of our current cases. Its increased transmissibility gives it an advantage that allows it to outcompete other variants. The increased transmissibility also makes it more difficult to control the virus using standard public health interventions like masks, social distancing, and ventilation. Adherence to those measures must be even higher to counter the variant's ease of spread. Fortunately, the performance of the vaccines authorized for use in the U.S. is not substantially impacted, and they still provide very high levels of protection against this variant.

B.1.1.7 is now joined by four others designated as "variants of concern" and several "variants of interest." The most concerning characteristic of these other variants is that they exhibit some degree of immune escape, meaning that vaccines and therapeutics may be somewhat less effective. Future variants may drift even further from the protection existing vaccines can provide, cause more severe illness, or impact diagnostic testing. These possibilities underscore the importance of careful surveillance and characterization of emerging variants. If we do need to update our vaccines or diagnostics to be a better match, we must know that as early as possible so we can begin that work before the variant becomes widespread. We must not again be unprepared.

The American Rescue Plan includes $1.7B for genomic surveillance, which the Biden Administration has announced will be spent on expanding sequencing, establishing Centers of Excellence in Genomic Epidemiology, and building a National Bioinformatics Infrastructure. These endeavors would be bolstered by the development of a national strategy that could enumerate near term and long-term priorities for advancing our genomic surveillance infrastructure, drawing on lessons from similar, successful efforts for influenza and foodborne illness. The development and implementation of the strategy could be led by the Department of Health and Human Services and supported by interagency and academic experts.

The American Rescue Plan also includes additional funds for biological research, expansion of the public health workforce, and a suite of other important public health initiatives that will improve our preparedness. Given that SARS-CoV-2 is likely to circulate both here and abroad for the foreseeable future, and in anticipation of the next viral threat, Congress should provide long-term, sustainable support for this expansion in public health infrastructure so that we will be in a position to better respond to the next threat.

Data Sharing

Timely collection and sharing of accurate, detailed public health data have long been a challenge during outbreaks. Public health data infrastructure is underdeveloped and out of date in many places around the world, including in the United States. Both the CARES Act and the American Rescue Plan contain funding for Centers for Disease Control and Prevention's (CDC) Data Modernization Initiative (DMI). DMI is an important plan to bring together state, tribal, local, and territorial public health jurisdictions as well as stakeholders from the public and private sectors to upgrade our national public health data infrastructure.

Genomic surveillance data should be included in the efforts of DMI. In some respects, sharing of viral genome data is more common than for other kinds of public health data. Although far from perfect, many scientists do share sequence data publicly, allowing others to analyze and learn from those data. Several public repositories exist and are widely used, including GISAID and GenBank. The GISAID repository includes over 1.4M submissions of SARS-CoV-2 sequences, including over 380,000 from the United States. Following the experience of the United Kingdom and the B.1.1.7 variant, sharing of sequence data has accelerated rapidly, and I expect that trend to continue.

However, several gaps in data sharing remain. Right now, most sharing is concentrated around individual sequences. But to determine whether a mutation or variant has clinical or public health consequences, we must be able to observe how the variant behaves in individuals and populations. To do that, researchers must know about the demographics, symptoms, clinical course and history, and outcomes of the person infected. Additional information about the circumstances of infection, including the number of secondary cases, is also valuable. For example, the United Kingdom was able to characterize the B.1.1.7 variant by analyzing case data linked with testing data. The New York City Department of Health and Mental Hygiene recently accomplished something similar with the B.1.526 variant, finding that it likely does not cause more severe disease.

The kind of data infrastructure that allows for analyses that combine sequence data with case data is not common in the United States. This gap limits our ability to understand whether new variants have changed in ways that are meaningful to public health, or whether they are simply benign variations. To remedy this, we should work toward the examples set by the United Kingdom and New York City by developing research partnerships between public health departments, laboratories and hospital systems, which is an effort that could be coordinated by the National Institutes of Health and CDC.

Modeling and Analytics

As we advance our genomic surveillance infrastructure, we should also further develop the modeling and analytics infrastructure that will allow us to make even better use of that data. Epidemiological modeling has played an important role both in the Covid-19 response and in previous epidemics, but that capability is not yet fully developed. With the exception of a few small groups within the Department of Health and Human Services, most modelers work in academia and volunteer to support the public health response when an urgent need arises. This arrangement is not well suited for either party.

The Federal government would benefit from a permanent capability, with infectious disease modelers working to advance the state of the science and support public health decision-making both between and during emergencies. Efforts along those lines are newly underway. The Biden Administration announced in National Security Directive-1 an intention to create a National Center for Epidemic Forecasting and Outbreak Analytics, and the American Rescue Plan appropriated $500M to CDC for disease forecasting and data modernization. These are promising steps towards modernizing our response capabilities, and I believe they will serve the nation well. Congress could help by appropriating annual funding for the forecasting center so that it can endure as a permanent program.

Future Preparedness

The challenges we face in setting up and maintaining genomic surveillance infrastructure are not unique to SARS-CoV-2. We have faced these challenges before with influenza surveillance, and we will at some point face them again with the next emerging pathogen. The lessons we learn and the investments we make to navigate through this crisis can also serve as an opportunity to fortify our preparedness and response infrastructure for other infectious disease threats that we face.

It is also in our interest to ensure that countries around the world are similarly equipped to conduct genomic surveillance in their communities. Although the United States is already achieving widespread vaccination which will slow circulation of the virus, that will not be the case in much of the world in the short or medium term. Continued transmission will facilitate the emergence of new variants, including potentially those that are not well matched for the vaccines. Bolstering surveillance globally will give warning to the world and allow medical countermeasures to be updated accordingly.

The United States could offer technical assistance and funding to other research and public health institutions that wish to develop and expand genomic surveillance.

In conclusion, although the currently circulating variants complicated our course through the spring months, we are now on track to regain control of the pandemic in the U.S. Continued vigilance to current and future variants is essential to ensuring that we maintain our encouraging trajectory. We must expand our genomic surveillance efforts domestically, and work with partners and allies abroad to ensure global coverage. The United States is a world leader in science and technology, and we have the opportunity, using those capabilities, to lead the world through the rest of the pandemic.

Discussion

Chairman FOSTER. Thank you. And at this point we will now begin our first round of questions. So the Chair will recognize himself for five minutes.

The first question is what I hope is sort of a simple question on the public health significance of new viral strains. Dr. Rivers, you note in your testimony that B.1.1.7 has gone on to become dominant in the United States, constituting perhaps 60 percent of our current cases. So my question is does that mean that if this variant had never existed that we would have 60 percent fewer cases in the United States today or is it more complicated than that? You know, should we think about these as, you know, each new strain is a whole new disease circulating in our population or are there things like, you know, cross-immunity that really muddy the picture here? And how should we think about this?

Dr. RIVERS. Yes, thank you for that question. It's not the case that we would have 60 percent fewer cases. What it means for a variant to be more transmissible is the tools we have, particularly around masking, distancing, ventilation, have to be adhered to even more closely in order to be effective because the virus passes more easily between people. The increased transmissibility is seen across a number of variants of concern and interest, and it makes it more difficult for the variants to be—the virus to be controlled and slowed.

Chairman FOSTER. OK. And so in the modeling do you model it as just one virus with a range of infectiousness or do you independently model the frequency of each strain in the population? I guess maybe that gets at my question.

Dr. RIVERS. There are several different approaches depending on the question you would like to answer. When producing a forecast, you would increase the infectiousness or the transmissibility, and so you would have a better sense of the new trajectory given the variant. If you would like to know how competing variants might unfold over time, it would be a different approach, but that is also a question that can be answered using modeling approaches.

Chairman FOSTER. Thank you. Dr. Abdool Karim, in your prepared testimony you gave a great overview of how the known variants have affected disease severity, transmissibility, and treatment efficacy, and as well as natural and vaccine-induced immunity. I think that addressed a lot of questions and concerns that I have as we see new variants pop up, but, you know, how—could you say a little bit about the difference between how variants will evolve before you have the population vaccinated or at least partially vaccinated versus after you've got a big part of the population vaccinated? You know, what fraction of the danger from a vaccine-induced mutation, what fraction of the woods are we out of in that—in regards to that?

Dr. ABDOOL KARIM. Thank you very much for that question. I think you're getting to one of the difficult areas that we don't have data, and so I what I'm going to tell you is speculation to some extent. What we understand now is immunocompromised individuals are playing an important role in the generation of variants, and so as the virus is spreading at a higher rate, we are enhancing the risk of seeing new variants.

When we have a vaccinated population, if a vaccinated individual or an individual who has had past infection or an individual who is receiving monoclonal antibodies has a virus that's evolving to create a variant, then that variant has a higher likelihood of escaping that immunity, and so that's our concern that as we get to higher levels of vaccination, the individuals who are immunocompromised that may lead to the emergence of new variants would be those at risk of creating variants with vaccine escape—ability to escape vaccine immunity.

Chairman FOSTER. And are we in a situation now at least in the United States that when we see what are called these breakthrough cases where you get vaccinated and nonetheless get COVID, are those of enough special interest that at least those are completely sequenced to see if we're seeing those as the source of new vaccine-resistant variants?

Dr. ABDOOL KARIM. So there are several programs underway, and many of the companies themselves as part of their clinical trials have been sequencing the viruses that constitute escape and also they want to measure the antibody levels at which escape is occurring. And the most recent published paper in the New England Journal of Medicine showed that two of the variants that had been sequenced and studied in detail that caused breakthrough infections, that they were variants with escaped mutations. So I think what we're going to see in breakthrough infections is a combination of normal viruses that are just escaping because immunity is low and others that have escaped mutations that enable them to bypass the immunity or at least partially bypass it.

Chairman FOSTER. And beautiful timing on ending your remarks as the timer goes to zero, and I will now recognize our Ranking Member, Mr. Obernolte, for five minutes.

Mr. OBERNOLTE. Well, thank you, Mr. Chairman, and thank you to all of our panelists. It's been a fascinating hearing.

I am very interested in what we can do as a Federal Government to change policy to make the process of identifying these variants and combating them more cost-effective and efficient. So, Dr. Grubaugh, I had a question for you because you talked about different policy changes that can be contemplated along those lines. And one of the things that you mentioned is giving data generators the first right to publish, which seems to me to be counterintuitive because, you know, wouldn't that slow the spread of information? We want to speed that up. So what could we do to help that?

Dr. GRUBAUGH. Yes, thank you for that question. It's a really complex area in public health. I think if data being generated by a public health lab and for the sole purpose of public health, then it makes sense just to make that free and open. In the United States we have a lot of data that are not being generated by public health labs but by academic labs that cost somewhere between, you know, $100 and $200 to sequence a virus genome. And when you have an academic lab whose first order of business is to support students and postdocs that need to publish to go on with their careers, if they're spending a lot of that time then giving the data away for free, then that can become problematic for those who actually need it.

Now, in my lab I am open data, open resource, open everything, and we're sort of in a privileged situation that we can make everything available. And if we get scooped on that, then we have other things to help make sure that our students get papers. But other people may not be in those privileged situations, especially in the low-resource countries where maybe they can't quite survive—a lab may not be able to survive having their data be poached by high- income countries. So it becomes a really complicated scenario, one that there's a national and global debate right now, and I hope that I answered your question.

Mr. OBERNOLTE. OK. Thank you. I would hope—we all would hope that at some point the greater good of sharing information to combat something which is an existential threat to humanity, you know, could prevail over parochial interests, and so anything that we can do as a government to stimulate that I think would be a good thing.

Dr. Karim, I found your testimony particularly interesting, and I wonder, you've testified that some variants such as the recent B.1.351 variant have proven to be problematic for some vaccines. And so, for example, vaccine efficacy of vaccines like AstraZeneca has been much lower whereas vaccines like the Pfizer vaccine and the Johnson & Johnson have not been as effective. So could you tell us a little bit more about why that is, why some vaccines are affected more than others and what we can do to improve that?

Dr. ABDOOL KARIM. Yes, thank you for that. So we don't fully understand why some vaccines are differentially affected and others are not, but I'll give you one of the possible reasons that might explain that. The mutation that occurs in position 484 is a particularly important mutation. Naturally when—in the pre-existing variants the position 484 has an amino acid that is negatively charged. The human cell at that point is also negatively charged, so the pre-existing variants have a bit of propulsion because of negative versus negative. However, when the mutation occurs, the virus becomes positively charged, so that enhances the ability of the virus to attach to the cell so it becomes more difficult for antibodies to displace it. It's what we refer to as electrostatic charge is impacting on that.

So the way in which the vaccine immunity can displace one that has more affinity is differential by the different vaccines, and that's probably the key explanation why the AstraZeneca vaccine is pretty much—has no efficacy against mild to moderate disease against B.1.351, whereas Pfizer at this point has 100 percent efficacy. And we only know this because both the trials were done in South Africa.

Mr. OBERNOLTE. Right. Well, thank you very much. I find that fascinating. One last question for Dr. Streiffer. A couple of our panelists have expressed the need for faster and less expensive whole-virus genome sequencing. What can we do as a Federal Government to make that faster and less expensive? Because it seems very central to our ability to fight these virus variants.

Dr. STREIFFER. You know, one example of that is really fascinating right now is actually wastewater testing. So a lot of the genetic information is actually coming from patient samples where you're tying that back to a specific patient. What's actually been very efficacious at least in high-income countries is the idea of actually doing pooled sampling from wastewater and then sequencing everything in that wastewater. And that gives you more of a shotgun approach to be able to understand everything that's coming out of the community and the ability to be able to detect variants well before they present through clinical patient testing. And it's got some limitations, but that's one way in which we could do something that's much cheaper.

I think Dr. Grubaugh also indicated some ways where you can actually design diagnostic tests that are simpler than the full genome sequencing but still allow you to sample variants in a way that gives you more visibility than the standard clinical testing, and that's a very important area to pursue.

Mr. OBERNOLTE. Well, great. Well, thank you. I've got about a dozen other questions, but I see my time's expired, so thank you to all of our panelists. And, Mr. Chairman, I yield back.

Chairman FOSTER. All right. It looks like we will have a shot at another—second set of questions if there—if interest is retained.

And I'll now recognize the Chairwoman of the Full Committee, Ms. Johnson, for five minutes.

Chairwoman JOHNSON. Thank you very much. Dr. Karim Abdool—Abdool Karim, the rollout of the vaccine to many and the much-needed light at the end of the tunnel of course we think after a year waiting and hoping that we've gotten there, the CDC has gradually upgraded its guidance on measures such as social distancing, mask wearing as vaccine uptake in the United States increases. However, we are still falling short of achieving herd immunity in this country and globally. How important are the behavioral measures in preventing the spread of the virus while we remain under the threshold for herd immunity? And what current state of science regarding the ability of the vaccinated individuals to asymptomatically infect nonvaccinated people?

Dr. ABDOOL KARIM. Thank you very much, Chairwoman Johnson. So let me try and answer the first question, which is that we vaccinate individuals for two reasons. The first is for individual benefit. I get a vaccine so I benefit in that I don't get severe disease or I don't get infected at all when I'm exposed. The second reason we vaccinate is we want population benefit. We want to slow the transmission of the virus. Now, we can only do that with vaccines if a person who's vaccinated does not transmit the virus because if a person who is vaccinated who gets infected then transmits the virus, then we undermine our ability to achieve herd immunity. So far, the preliminary data—and it's pretty—it's very preliminary— suggests that transmission rates are dropped in individuals who are vaccinated, but we do not yet have definitive evidence because those studies are hard to do.

The second issue—the second question you asked me is about how important it is that we maintain our nonpharmaceutical prevention measures while we are vaccinating. It is critical because vaccines on their own are not able to achieve herd immunity or to slow transmission on their own. We do need to maintain those.

When we start nearing levels of herd immunity with vaccine coverage only, I think what we will then see is a change in the number of restrictions that will be required, and many of the individual restrictions will be replaced by broader restrictions such as avoiding mass gatherings where the risk is high, but for the individual restrictions, we can expect that some of those will be eased, and the CDC has been doing that in a systematic, slow way at the moment.

Chairwoman JOHNSON. Thank you very much. Mr. Chairman, I yield back.

Chairman FOSTER. Thank you, and I will now recognize our colleague from Florida, Mr. Posey, for five minutes.

Mr. POSEY. Thank you very much, Chairman Foster and Ranking Member Obernolte, for holding this hearing.

Discussing the variants of COVID–19 is very important to our work of defeating this virus and understanding its dangers and history. Dr. Streiffer, in 2003 it appears the first SARS epidemic, SARS-CoV, was beginning to spread, and the virus was mutating rapidly as it adapted to humans. But it appears once it became more contagious, it became more stable and stopped mutating so quickly.

COVID–19 or SARS-CoV–2, appears to have been remarkably stable since it first emerged in 2019 in Wuhan. It never appears to have had the same period of rapid mutation that was seen in the 2003 SARS outbreak. Each witness obviously is very interested in the variants, but I wonder if we are as curious about the missing links for earlier variants of COVID–19 that we would have expected to have seen just after the emergence of a new virus. Can staff bring my pictures up now?

[Slide follows (next page):]

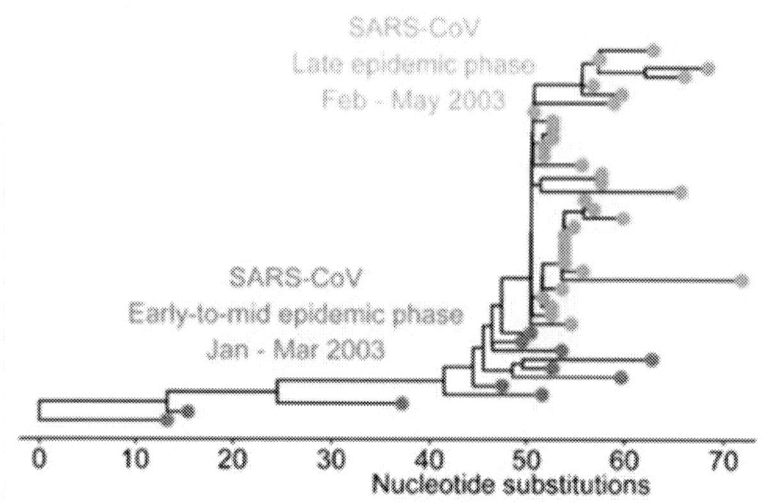

Figure 1.

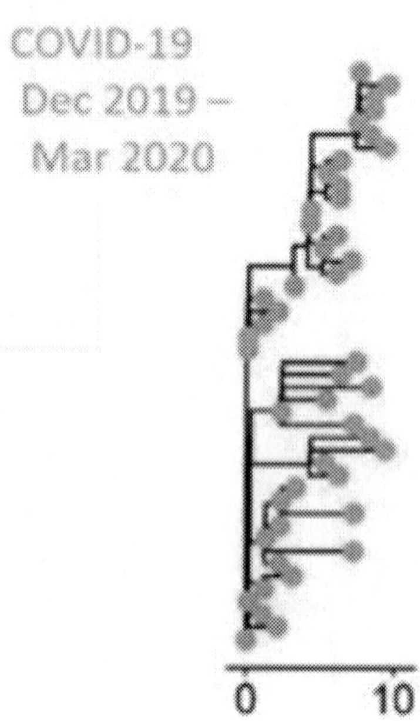

Figure 2.

Mr. POSEY. This is from a preprint paper, and figure 1 shows mutations in early stage SARS in blue and then the late-stage SARS in yellow. Figure 2 shows the mutations in COVID–19. Bigger spaces between those dots would appear to this layperson to indicate greater mutations in the virus. And obviously, the two figures are very different from each other, and in fact the red COVID, COVID–19 looks a lot more like the yellow late-stage SARS. The original SARS is known to be a nationally emerging virus, and it mutated rapidly when it did emerge. COVID–19 on the other hand did not have the same rapid mutations. So my question, Dr. Streiffer, based on your expertise, how would you explain why figure 2 does not have the early mutations that we see in figure 1? Dr. STREIFFER. So just to jump in—and sorry, I apologize, I moving screens around so I can actually see the figure. I'm actually paying attention. So I think virus evolution is always a careful balance between trying to infect the host, replicate, and do that in a way which is efficient but not actually kill the host. And one of the things that you'll find is that vaccine—viruses rather are actually too aggressive they cause too much fatality and will actually damp out very quickly, so you do see an enormous amount of difference in the rate at which viruses mutate and the patterns that you see in those mutations.

And I think that's reflected here. I think these are both natural viruses. I think the difference in the mutation rates is a reflection of the different epidemiology, the way in which the initial pandemic's played out, and then just the natural differences in the virus.

And Dr. Abdool Karim and Dr.—excuse me, I'm going to get my name wrong—Dr. Grubaugh could probably comment very eloquently on this if they'd like to follow up with that, although, of course, it's the Member's prerogative.

Mr. POSEY. I'd be delighted for the follow-up. Thank you. I yield.

Chairman FOSTER. Thank you. The gentleman has yielded his time for—

Mr. POSEY. I was going to yield to the witness to answer that Dr. Streiffer recommended.

Dr. GRUBAUGH. I can answer for a minute. So, one, each virus is a little bit different, and especially when we have viruses that emerge from animals and to people that they're at different stages of being able to adapt and spread within people. And so there's— it's always hard to compare apples to apples when you have different events that are happening.

Also, evolution is not just dependent on adapting to the host. There's other things in play such as the re-transmission, some other inherent factors, the types of therapeutics that are used, so it's a really complicated factor.

And I would say that with SARS CoV–2 we did see early adaptation to humans. We had the D614G mutation that rapidly spread around the world, and then now we are seeing the emergence of many new variants that are happening. And also just to say that the pandemic with SARS-CoV–2 is really unprecedented in terms of the number of infections. It's evolutionary patterns with the emergence of several variants that have many mutations that are acquired in a very short period that I would just say it's very difficult to compare this to really anything else because we haven't seen anything quite like this.

Mr. POSEY. Thank you very much. Mr. Chairman, thank you. I yield back.

Chairman FOSTER. Thank you. And, yes, the—I believe the gentleman's line of questioning touched on a very important issue, which is trying to understand what we can about the origins of this virus. And, you know, this is a subject of very serious scientific debate among serious scientists about what constitutes evidence in various directions. This Subcommittee on Investigations and Oversight does intend to have a hearing on the origins of the SARS- CoV–2 virus in the near future.

And I will now recognize our colleague from California, Dr. Bera, for five minutes.

Mr. BERA. Thank you, Chairman Foster.

I know that, you know, that tracking variants and making sure we're data sharing is something that we've been incredibly interested in—along with Senator Tammy Baldwin from Wisconsin, we introduced the Tracking COVID–19 Variants Act asking for $2 billion to go to CDC. We were able to get $1.75 billion into the American Rescue Plan, so hopefully, that's a first step, as well as indicating to the CDC to talk about the issue that I know—I think we've talked to Dr. Rivers about data sharing and how we, you know, link public health and academia and data sharing.

I'm going to put my doctor hat on and just, you know, when I think about the variants that we're seeing in India, you know, also some of the variants that we're seeing in Michigan or some of the cases that we're seeing, it does seem like, you know, younger people are now being infected more rapidly, as well as being hospitalized. And I don't know if that's just epidemiology that younger folks are less vaccinated and thus are susceptible, and maybe, Dr. Karim, you know, since you're on the frontline in South Africa, you could tell us what you're seeing on the ground in terms of hospitalizations of who is being infected right now.

Dr. ABDOOL KARIM. Thank you for the question. Yes, you're quite right. It's a matter of epidemiology. And we saw that certainly in the second wave in Brazil, South Africa, and in India, that in the second wave, because the virus has a higher transmissibility, it infects a lot more people quickly. The number of younger people in those populations is high, and so even though it's a smaller fraction that will actually get to a hospital, so many of them became infected that disproportionately there were larger numbers of young people in hospitals, so it's just a function of the way in which the rapid transmissibility infects such a high proportion of young people that we begin to see more young people in hospitals. And that's been described quite well in all three settings. And it's a similar issue with the B.1.1.7 variant, that it causes many young people to get infected, so that's why disproportionately we start seeing more young people in hospital. You're quite right.

Mr. BERA. And, you know, for any of the panelists, as we think about that then, you know, I think many of us in the medical community were surprised that India, Sub-Saharan Africa, et cetera, weren't severely impacted in the first wave a year ago, and some of us thought that, well, it's a younger population so they had sub-clinical infections, et cetera. Now our concern is that we're seeing these variants spread more rapidly with younger population, what this may do in Sub-Saharan Africa that also speaks to a younger population. Is that a legitimate concern? And, you know, obviously we're seeing the overwhelming infections in India. And how should we—outside of rapidly getting vaccinations to these populations, how else should we think about it? And, again, I'm happy to let— or Dr. Karim, if you want to answer that one as well.

Dr. ABDOOL KARIM. Sure, I'll start with an answer. I have spent the last several months trying to answer that question. That's because we all predicted that Africa would have a really severe epidemic, but it didn't come to pass, and so there was some hypotheses that were proposed. And I have looked at nine of the different hypotheses, including temperature, including age, and so on.

I think in summary I have found that there is no specific protection that Africans have. There's nothing in their lifestyle, there's nothing that they've got genetically that gives them any protection that I have been able to find.

What is most clear is that the young populations that we see in Africa, the very small fractions of the population that are above 60 means that a large number of people who are getting infected are getting infected asymptomatically, and so the reporting has been— you know, they don't report those cases because they don't know about those cases. In addition, most of the countries in Africa went into very severe lockdowns initially, so that's why the first waves weren't that bad. But now they're being caught in the second wave and the variants where many countries in Africa have much more severe epidemics. So variants, age, and implementing nonpharmaceutical interventions early played that role in why I think Africa did not see a severe epidemic. And I'm sure my colleagues may have something to add. Thank you.

Mr. BERA. I see I'm out of time. Hopefully, we'll have that second round of questions.

Chairman FOSTER. And we plan to. And now, despite the fact that he is not a doctor but merely holds a master's degree in biochemical engineering, the Chair will now recognize our colleague from Illinois, Mr. Casten, for five minutes.

Mr. CASTEN. Oh, you're far too kind. It's nice to be one of the non-nerds in this group.

I really want to thank you all for being here. Thank you to our Chairman for pulling this hearing together.

The—Dr. Abdool Karim, I want to start with you and I think just give us a chance to have a little bit of a—just a few quick public service announcements. The—you know, we are fortunately going from a point in our country where we shifted from having more demand than supply for vaccine to, you know, starting to see the opposite and, you know, daily doses administered have fallen off in the last month or so and starting to sort of get to that harder more vaccine-hesitant community.

I want to start with a public service announcement of my own. My 16-year-old daughter is getting her second dose in two weeks, and my 14-year-old daughter has just registered for her first dose tomorrow, so what's good for us is good for—and hopefully everyone will follow.

But, Dr. Abdool Karim—and you mentioned this before, but just a couple quick yes or noes. To the best of your knowledge are the Moderna, Pfizer, and J&J vaccines currently available to Americans effective at preventing the worst aspects of COVID–19?

Dr. ABDOOL KARIM. Yes.

Mr. CASTEN. To your knowledge are they all generally safe?

Dr. ABDOOL KARIM. Yes.

Mr. CASTEN. To your knowledge are they broadly effective against all of the common variants of COVID–19 that are circulating in the United States?

Dr. ABDOOL KARIM. I can't answer that exactly, but they are effective against most of the common variants. They haven't been tested against, for example, the Indian variant yet, the variant in India.

Mr. CASTEN. OK. Well, there's—is there any good reason for any American, unless their doctor tells them otherwise, not to go get a vaccine?

Dr. ABDOOL KARIM. No.

Mr. CASTEN. OK. Well, that's an easy one.

Let me then move on to something a little bit more deep in the weeds. And you alluded to some of this in your conversation with Chairwoman Johnson. Early on I think we were all concerned about what is the likelihood of asymptomatic spread and how do we know about that and how do we think through that. Have you seen anything in the data to suggest that the risk of asymptomatic thread is—excuse me—asymptomatic spread is substantially different between vaccinated and nonvaccinated populations?

Dr. ABDOOL KARIM. We don't have empiric data, so I'm going to speculate based on what we have been seeing in terms of the viral load that's in the swabs that are taken from the nose. When we look at the swab—the amount of virus that's in the swab, vaccinated individuals who do get infected have lower levels of the virus in those swabs. So we would think that that translates into lower transmission, but I don't have clinical evidence. That laboratory evidence is certainly suggestive that vaccination means lower levels of transmission.

Mr. CASTEN. And what about for folks who have, you know, tested positive for COVID and may have developed some degree of natural immunity? How would you put that population in amongst the vaccinated versus nonvaccinated?

Dr. ABDOOL KARIM. So individuals who have had prior infection generally have some level of protection to new infections even if they are variants. And the level of protection that's provided is at this point most likely in terms of the severity of infection, so they may be able to transmit, but we think that they get less severe disease. The empiric data for that is still preliminary. Only—there's only one study I've seen it, and that's of a small number that suggests that.

But in terms of transmission, an individual who's been infected gets reinfection, we don't know about their risk of transmission. I can't answer that question.

Mr. CASTEN. So I—and I realize I may be getting into small subsets of data, but if—you talked about viral loading as being your sort of estimate of why this might change. If you have experienced COVID but not been vaccinated versus experienced COVID and have been vaccinated, is there a difference in the viral loading of those two populations? I mean, what I'm trying to get at is do we expand herd immunity more greatly by making sure that even if you've had a bad case of COVID and you still get vaccinated, do you reduce your risk of asymptomatic spread at least theoretically?

Dr. ABDOOL KARIM. There's a big difference. If we look at vaccinated individuals, especially when they've been vaccinated with an mRNA vaccine, the antibody levels are really high. They are extremely high. They are at the highest levels that we see with natural infection, as opposed to natural infection where the antibodies are much lower. And when you deal with variants, higher antibodies are really important, higher levels of these antibodies, so there's no question that vaccination is a big advantage compared to natural infection in terms of risk of reinfection.

Also, that when you've had natural infection, if you've had asymptomatic natural infection, the antibodies disappear quite early, within three, to four, five months, and so we see lower levels of antibodies with asymptomatic infections in natural infections, but with vaccines, it's consistent. Everybody gets high levels of antibodies.

Mr. CASTEN. It's fascinating. And I'm unfortunately out of time. I have more questions, but I really appreciate your time. I yield back.

Chairman FOSTER. Thank you. And I will now recognize our colleague from Colorado, Mr. Perlmutter, for five minutes.

Mr. PERLMUTTER. Thank you, Dr. Foster. And I guess I want to start with a question that was posed early on in this process, and that was sort of Sweden's approach toward herd immunity by, you know, just sort of going on with their lives compared to surrounding Scandinavian countries. And this is to the whole panel. You know, I haven't seen much in the news about Sweden and its herd immunity and whether or not it's facing any new challenges given these variations. So, Dr. Rivers, why don't I start with you if you have any—or anybody who wants to jump in on that one.

Dr. RIVERS. Sure. I can't speak to the latest situation in Sweden as I haven't followed up on their current status, but I will note that their early strategy of allowing the infection to spread in hopes of achieving naturally acquired herd immunity was changed over time, and they did go on to adapt more restrictive measures in order to slow the spread because they saw that their hospitals were becoming overwhelmed. And so I think that our early perception of how Sweden managed the pandemic was something that evolved to look more in line with the measures that many other countries took. But I'll see if any of my colleagues know the latest on Sweden.

Mr. PERLMUTTER. Anybody else?

Dr. ABDOOL KARIM. I can perhaps just comment briefly. I just did a webinar with Anders Tegnell, who is the chief COVID scientist in Sweden, my equivalent there, and he went with this initial approach, which is—actually was promoted by a group of scientists in—across the oceans both in the United States and the U.K. under something called the Great Barrington Declaration. And their hypothesis was if you let the virus run wild in younger populations, natural infection will provide immunity and herd immunity. Well, it's been shown now that that simply is not true, that in fact what happens is when you end up with large numbers of infections like that, the older people do get infected and you get the situation of high numbers of death. And Sweden saw that and so had to make those changes. And Sweden, by the way, still doesn't promote mask wearing, but that's a separate discussion. It's not related to this.

Mr. PERLMUTTER. All right, thank you. Yes, I mean, what—you saw the initial, you know, reports was, you know, Norway had a much smaller incidence than Sweden as Sweden was trying to, you know, develop herd immunity. They were having a lot sicker people and deaths compared to their next-door neighbor. So—OK. Thank you.

Now I'm going to ask more personal questions because, Dr. Rivers, I'm one of those 32 million who was infected. And, you know, my curiosity is more in these variations. You know, we've talked about two things, how transmissible it is and how severe the new variations may be. So, you know, one thing we haven't talked and I'd ask the Chair and the Ranking Member that we also take a look at sort of the long-term effects of this disease. And, you know, we do know that there are issues that linger. So in terms of the severity of some of these new, more transmissible viruses, what are we seeing in terms of the effect on people's health? Is there something that, say, in the South African variation is more dangerous in terms of health or is it just because it's more transmissible? So, Dr. Grubaugh, why don't you—I don't know if you want to jump in on that or if that's something you've been thinking about or anybody else.

Dr. GRUBAUGH. I'll just quickly start, and I believe Dr. Rivers probably has some points to make here, too. There is some data from the U.K. that would indicate that the B.1.1.7 variant can cause more severe disease. It's not just more transmissible. It's a really difficult thing to actually answer because when you're— there's—you know, what has the most impact on disease is actually host factors, age, comorbidities. These sorts of things impact whether or not you're going to be—you know, have more severe disease or not, much more than the virus. So the virus could have some small impacts on that, but we need really large studies to be able to measure these sort of small changes.

Mr. PERLMUTTER. OK. Dr. Rivers?

Dr. RIVERS. Thank you. I'll just add that there are three levels of variant classification in the United States, variants of interest, variants of concern, and the third is a variant of high consequence. And the variant that causes more severe disease would be classified as a variant of high consequence. There are currently no variants that carry that designation, and so that's not something that is currently circulating or has been identified.

Mr. PERLMUTTER. Thank you. My time is expired. I yield back.

Chairman FOSTER. Well, thank you. And at this point we will now begin our second round of questions, and the Chair will recognize himself for five minutes.

Dr. Streiffer, it was I guess about a year ago last week the Science Committee held its first roundtable about the Federal research enterprise and its response to COVID–19. And we talked about the natural—National Virtual Biotechnology Laboratory with Michelle Buchanan of Oak Ridge. And at the time NVBL was only a few weeks old, and now with a year of experience behind you, you know, there are serious efforts to consider a permanent reauthorization of the NVBL both by—on the part of our former colleague, now Senator Ben Ray Lujan, as well as efforts in the House. And so with that year of experience behind you, what are the observations that you might have about the best practices on how to coordinate all of the diverse Federal capabilities that were brought together in the NVBL?

Dr. STREIFFER. Thank you, Dr. Foster. It's a very good question. I think some of the lessons learned from that is that the coordination across the 17 laboratories through a central body was actually very effective. And coordinating that directly with the Department of Energy and then with each of the agencies that's been involved in the national response is crucially important. And I think one thing that's very gratifying is the increased level of coordination that we're seeing over the last several months in the Nation's response to COVID–19.

I think also very importantly is that the National Virtual Biotechnology Laboratory created a model that was very flexible, very adaptive, and very fast to respond to the issues, much different than we often think of the national response framework, particularly when research and development is concerned where those timescales are quite long. And with that adaptability I think we're able to quickly pivot to the most important problems at hand, maintain a focus on issues that they—as they developed and move on from issues like designing new ventilators as it became apparent that those were not going to be as of a concern as they initially appeared to be.

Chairman FOSTER. Thank you. And I guess my next question is for any of the witnesses that might want to get to it. Do we really have a complete picture of how this disease spreads? You know, is it—for example, if it's airborne, is it a few large droplets that someone sprays at you while we're talking and gets inhaled deeply into the lungs or is it the ambient concentration of very small viral particles when you walk into a bar that's just had people in it for hours? How important is direct ingestion of the virus compared to inhalation both through the nose and directly into lungs? You know, what's the model here? Is it every virus that gets into your respiratory tract has the same probability, or are there certain configurations that are dangerous? What's understood about that?

Dr. RIVERS. I can perhaps start. This is one of the areas of our understanding of the virus that has changed substantially over time. We—particularly because it's difficult when people are in close contact to determine which mode of transmission was actually the one that infected them, but there's a growing understanding that the virus can buildup in the air and that crowded environments, even if you are not within 6 feet of someone, can be particularly risky. On the other hand, our perception of fomite transmission or contaminated services has gone down in the list and it is no longer considered one of the primary modes of transmission. And I would put even below that ingestion. So airborne and respiratory are—excuse me, airborne and droplet transmission are at the top of the list.

Chairman FOSTER. Any other comments? You know, one of the reasons I bring it up is that the British are now apparently going to go ahead and do experiments in controlled human infection where they're going to be testing the efficacy directly of several candidate vaccines, which is one of the applications to very quickly get accurate measurements of the efficacy, you know, months faster than you can with standard clinical trials but also to get a better understanding of the methods of spread. And this is one of the tools that, you know, many people wish were available. You know, had we understood the role—the small role of fomites compared to inhalations on—early in the pandemic, we would be in a position to save hundreds of thousands of lives. If you can have some questions answered through those sort of experiments of direct human infection, what are the questions you'd really like to have answered in that kind of thing, or do you think that they won't really in the end be that useful?

Dr. ABDOOL KARIM. Perhaps I'll just add a quick comment if I might. I think Dr. Rivers really captured the issues quite well. We were initially taken with the wide spread of infection on the cruise liners, and we thought that fomites were important, but now it's becoming clearer and certainly in mice experiments, mice in different cages are infecting each other, showing the importance of aerosol transmissions, the very small droplets that carry the virus. But I think the droplet spread I think still remains probably, you know, the most important or, together with aerosols, is the most important. So I think that still remains our main focus, that having direct infection is still quite important, and then aerosols and then fomites being much more less important.

Chairman FOSTER. Well, thank you. And if there is some best state-of-the-knowledge document that you could forward to our offices, it would be very valuable for any of the witnesses because it's—it matters a lot for policy obviously.

My time is up. I will now recognize the Ranking Member, Mr. Obernolte, for five minutes.

Mr. OBERNOLTE. Thank you, Mr. Chairman. This has been a fascinating discussion, and I want to continue the discussion along the lines of our ability to combat this kind of crisis in the future because I think that when the dust settles, we put this crisis behind us, and we do a postmortem, we're going to realize how extraordinarily fortunate we were that the level of antigenic drift of COVID–19 was not higher. So to prepare ourselves for the future I think we need to really focus on the lessons that we've learned here, on how the virus is transmitted, and, more importantly, how it mutates and how those mutations affect immune escape and the ability of the vaccines we develop to react to it.

So to any of our panelists that want to comment on this, how can the U.S. Government catalyze that kind of spread of information? Because I think it's going to be vital to our future ability to respond to these kind of crises.

Dr. STREIFFER. So I'll jump in here. I'd also add in addition to that one of the things we need to do is a much better job of what you would refer to as international zoonotic surveillance. So by the best scientific knowledge available to us, this disease came to mankind originally from bats. What we need to do is a much better job of understanding the viruses that are out there that could cross the species barrier, sample those, understand their threat, and track them as they move through potentially the wildlife populations and into contact with humans. That's something we need to invest much more in globally.

Dr. GRUBAUGH. I'll jump in here, too, with this question. So of course we—you know, the hope is that, you know, with continued evolution and, you know, some level of transmission of this virus likely for years to come, that we don't have significant antigenic drift where this would significantly impact our vaccines, but I think we need to be prepared for that worst-case scenario. And the goal here would then be to sequence, you know, first, you know, as many of the vaccine breakthroughs as possible. I think these are really important to do, and then maintaining this general surveillance that we have on a yearly basis similar to what has already been done for flu for a long time to help inform vaccines. I think this is going to be one of the most critical areas as we go forward and have some level where there's always going to be some pockets of transmission probably at least for the next several years and being able to stay on top of how the virus is evolving and not having to respond from behind like we did starting at the beginning of this year.

Mr. OBERNOLTE. Right. Well, thank you very much to everyone, and let me restate my opinion that more funding into this kind of research is vitally important for us. I mean, it might be a case of existential survival for us as a species to make sure that we understand the threat that's out there and the way that we as governments and as a world health community can respond to it. So thank you very much, Mr. Chairman, and thank you to our witnesses. I yield back.

Chairman FOSTER. Thank you. And we'll now recognize Dr. Bera for five minutes.

Mr. BERA. Great, thank you. You know, maybe this is a question for Dr. Karim. When we talk about the vaccines, obviously, we talk about the efficacy of the vaccines. But each of the vaccines, including AstraZeneca, seem to be efficacious at preventing severe illness, hospitalization, and death. Is that a correct statement?

Dr. ABDOOL KARIM. Yes, against the D614G variant, pretty much all the vaccines seem to be doing quite well in preventing severe disease both in the clinical trials but more importantly in the real world data that's now being collected.

Mr. BERA. OK. So, you know, while the AstraZeneca vaccine is not as effective at preventing illness necessarily, it's still, you know, an important component of our arsenal as we try to vaccinate the entire world. Is that——

Dr. ABDOOL KARIM. So that's a little bit more difficult. So the studies that have been done with other variants, not the D614G variant, so if you take, for example—I'll just—to simplify just focus on the variant that was first described in South Africa by us, the B.1.351, that variant, the studies that have been done only included younger people in South Africa with the AstraZeneca vaccine, so we know it doesn't work for mild and moderate infections in the South African setting against the B.1.351. The problem is we don't know if it prevents and ameliorates severe disease because there were no severe infections in the study itself.

And so there's only indirect evidence. There's only speculation and, you know, using laboratory evidence to suggest that maybe it will protect against severe disease, but there is no clinical evidence. And so on that basis——

Mr. BERA. If I were to ask Dr. Rivers or any of the other panelists—because obviously there's real-world evidence. You know, many people have gotten the AstraZeneca vaccine. Are we seeing those that have been vaccinated with AZ, let's say, in the United Kingdom and Britain being hospitalized or dying? Again, I have not seen anecdotal evidence that folks that have been vaccinated with the AZ even in places where there's a high prevalence of variants ending up dying? Is that—again, you know, Dr. Rivers?

Dr. RIVERS. I'm not sure that there is data available describing what Dr. Abdool Karim is sharing about the clinical evidence, but there are many places in the world where the immune escape variants are not circulating. The B.1.351 to my knowledge is not prevalent in many countries, and so the AZ and similar platforms would still have value there.

Mr. BERA. OK. Shifting—a question that's, you know, certainly— that I've been pondering since the beginning of the pandemic is, you know, when I think about how hard New York City was hit and then I think about Tokyo and how Japan, you know, approached the pandemic, you know, with the older population in Japan with mass transit systems, et cetera, you know, it was quite remarkable that they escaped, you know, at least in the first phase, you know, a similar impact that New York City potentially possessed. And I would just be curious, again, you know, this is the opinions of folks, obviously, mask wearing has a significant impact and culturally, you know, that's not taboo in Japan, and that was an issue—you know, the politics around mask wearing in the United States clearly had some impact. But is there a cross-immunity? You know, Japan, Korea, other places probably did get exposed to SARS and other coronaviruses in previous pandemics, and I would just be curious, you know, why Japan or, you know, or some of the Asian nations, you know, skirted the first phase of this, whereas we got hit quite hard? Maybe Dr. Rivers or any of the panelists.

Dr. RIVERS. The number of people infected by the SARS pandemic in 2003 was quite small, and so I don't expect it would contribute meaningfully to population immunity really anywhere in the world. Several of the Asian countries were much swifter and more aggressive in their response with—after the emergence of the novel coronavirus, and I think that contributed to their success. Japan focused very heavily on contact tracing, particularly backwards contact tracing, and I think that lent itself well to early containment. South Korea was also very successful, Singapore. They focused very heavily on diagnostic testing. They had a testing volume many times over what the United States was doing at the time, which allowed them to find cases. And so the overarching lesson for me is that we need to be prepared to respond very quickly even before we really can characterize and feel confident that the threat is severe. If you fall behind, it's very difficult to catch up. Mr. BERA. And the impact of wearing masks in Asia versus the United States?

Dr. RIVERS. Certainly in many countries in Asia after the 2003 pandemic it became common to wear masks in the community, and I—and many countries not only did they have them stockpiled but people had them in their homes, and I think that was very helpful as well.

Mr. BERA. Great. I'll yield back.

Chairman FOSTER. Yes, thank you. And I should also say in my one experience on Tokyo subways, it was very crowded but people were not talking, and I have never been on a New York subway where there weren't multiple people mouthing off in various ways. And we will now recognize our colleague, Representative Posey, for five minutes.

Mr. POSEY. Thank you very much, Mr. Chairman.

The thing that alarmed me the most about COVID–19 in the very beginning is when we got our first TV reports. They said the damage to your lungs from this virus is unlike any others that we've ever seen before, and it will not heal itself. It's irreversible damage like neurological damage. You might stop it from progressing, but you can never reverse all the damage it's done. Of course, we've heard an awful lot of people have fully recovered.

I remember talking to NASA (National Aeronautics and Space Administration) Administrator Jim Bridenstine right after he got tested, and he was sick at the time he got tested. And he said the doctor called him and said what do you want first, the good news or the bad news? And he said, well, give me the good news. He said, well, you don't have COVID. He said, well, then what's the bad news? He said, well, you've got the other virus that's already killed 80,000 people. But I guess that other virus didn't kill anybody after COVID came out. I guess it was stopped in its tracks. I was wondering, Dr. Streiffer, if the answer to my question that I asked before, you mentioned that you would expect to see this natural evolution, yet no one has presented any evidence of the evolution of COVID in animals or humans prior to the December 2019 outbreak. What do you make of that?

Dr. STREIFFER. I think there's a general understanding about the time that COVID–19 emerged as a disease in China. You know, as we've discussed previously, I think there's still some details about its origin that we don't quite understand. But I think the path of the virus upon its initial detection and its propagation around the world has followed more or less what we would expect for a virus that at some level has hit that sweet spot of being just infectious enough to spread, dangerous enough that it's caught our attention, but not so dangerous to kill so many hosts that it tamps itself down.

So, again, I would respectfully ask the Member to perhaps call on Dr. Rivers or Dr. Karim or Dr. Grubaugh to add some additional perspective on this. But I think we're seeing a progression in the genetic evolution of the virus under the pressures that we would expect from both nonpharmaceutical interventions and how the vaccines are taking hold that is within the spectrum that we would anticipate as scientists.

Mr. POSEY. You know, I've had a lot of—and I'll direct this to Dr. Karim. I've had a lot of constituents question about taking the vaccination. You know, you mentioned a blanket statement absolutely everybody should and there's no good reason for anybody not to, but I've had people, well, what if my sister has pneumonia? I mean, should she take it then? Well, I mean, common sense would dictate no, but I'm not a doctor, and there are people that have contacted my office, we've had bad outcomes from vaccines before, and I'm sure you're probably familiar with that. And I've just told people talk to your physician about it. Your physician knows best of all if you should get it, and I've had some sort of vaccine—hey, my physician said not to do it. Well, I'm not going to argue with your physician about that.

You know, I'm aware of the vaccine injury trust fund. I don't know if you all are familiar with it or not, but when people make these statements that vaccines are 100 percent safe for everybody without exception, end of subject, you're an idiot if you don't get vaccinated, the public is in large part unaware of the vaccine injury trust fund, which is very hard to access, has a 2-year statute of limitations on it. Most pediatricians tell people they're crazy if they think their kids were injured or whatever. That vaccine injury trust fund has paid out $4.5 billion and hasn't paid for a lot of the common bad outcomes that people suffer. So, Dr. Karim, just your thoughts briefly on that?

Dr. ABDOOL KARIM. Yes, thank you for that question. So I think all vaccines carry some side effects, and so that's part and parcel of what we live with. It's a question of the benefits and risks. In my own clinic I have had two severe reactions, one of which was very severe. The patient hospitalized, demyelinating disease, and she happened to have lupus, systemic lupus erythematosus. So she has a history of this kind of problem, and she didn't do well with the vaccine. I'm not sure if she actually got COVID, you know, she would probably also have quite a severe form of COVID, but we can never say that vaccines are 100 percent safe. There will always be those effects, and we've seen with some of the vaccines, clotting disorders. We've seen a range of others—I see them in my clinic. But I also see all of the many patients with severe COVID in my clinic, and I've got, you know, several patients with long COVID, and I can't tell you how debilitating it is. I'd rather you put up with the side effects and, you know, the antigenicity of the vaccine than have to deal with long COVID. I watch it and I shudder.

Mr. POSEY. I see my time is up. Mr. Chairman, thank you very much. I yield back.

Chairman FOSTER. Thank you. And we will—finally, we will now recognize our colleague from Colorado, Mr. Perlmutter, for five minutes.

Mr. PERLMUTTER. Thanks. And what Dr. Karim was just talking about is—I think should be another panel on the long-term effects of this and the potential costs associated with it because they do exist, and they are debilitating and—for some.

So my question is—let's start with Dr. Karim. When you were talking about immunoescape, you also mentioned people who are immunocompromised were more likely to have the virus do an immunoescape. And so can you tell me what you mean by immunocompromised and then the immunoescape? I wasn't quite sure I got it.

Dr. ABDOOL KARIM. Sure. So when the person gets naturally infected, the body's immune system goes through three steps—well, there's many steps but just to make it simple, an innate immunity and then you get the B cells and the T cells responding, so those are the three parts. In somebody who is immunocompromised, let's say, somebody who has got cancer and is on immunosuppressive treatment, they don't follow those three steps, and so they can't bring the virus under quick control. Their innate response is first and foremost your first line of defense, and it brings the virus under some control quickly. So if you don't do that, the virus continues to replicate for months and months and months. And it remains viable all those months. And as it's replicating in the presence of antibodies against the virus, the virus itself will start mutating. So these antibodies are not killing the virus, but they are exposing this virus to what it needs to bypass. And so that's what the problem is.

And so when we see—there's a superb paper in the New England Journal of Medicine, and that paper shows in the cancer patient over a period of four months how the virus systematically evolves and changes itself to bypass the immune response. And so that's— those are the individuals seem to be an important group in creating these shifts where these new variants are emerging.

Mr. PERLMUTTER. Thank you. Anybody else? Or I'm happy to yield back to the Chair. I appreciate that answer. Dr. Grubaugh?

Dr. GRUBAUGH. Yes, I'll just add onto that. I think Dr. Abdool Karim's explanation was really fantastic. And from the evolutionary perspective when we see natural infections and transmission so acute infections and then you transmit to somebody else and you look at that over the course of four months or so, there's about one to two mutations that are incorporated into the virus per month. When we look at some of these long infections, either, you know, some level of immunocompromised, obviously, that's a huge sort of range of things, it could be somebody who had an organ transplant and they're on immunosuppressive drugs, it could get somebody who has AIDS, cancer, right, a lot of different ways. And when the immune system can't quickly just clear the virus and it's left in some sort of middle state, it provides a great selective advantage. And that's where we see these new mutations rising quicker than what we would have in just natural—you know, a person-to-person acute transmission.

The other thing that happens that we see is the virus responds really quickly to some of our drugs and monoclonal antibodies. And if they're not completely suppressing the virus, it gives an opportunity again for the virus to adapt. So we end up with these—during these prolonged infections in immunocompromised individuals we see some of those exact same mutations that we find in variants of interest and variants of concern.

And so one of the hypotheses is that some of these variants that all of a sudden acquire, you know, 10, 20 different mutations and many of those occurring in the spike protein where we're really concerned with, that some period of time later in infection when you have the viremia that goes up, they might be transmitting to other people, and therefore, you have these sort of jumps then of viruses that are adapted to humans. I mean, that's one of the hypotheses here. And then, you know, these events are still probably pretty rare overall, but when you have millions and millions and millions of infections that have happened that—and these jump and then they're more transmissible, I think that's one of the explanations for what we're seeing for the rise of many of these variants.

Mr. PERLMUTTER. Thank you to this panel. You guys really are— have been educating me, and I appreciate it. I yield back to the Chair.

Chairman FOSTER. Thank you. And before we bring this hearing to a close, I want to myself thank our witnesses for testifying before the Committee today. And for those Members and witnesses with time, at the close of the hearing we can just hang around for some informal discussions as we often do following in-person hearings.

The record will remain open for two weeks for additional statements from the Members and for any additional questions that the Committee may ask of the witnesses. And this hearing is now adjourned.

[Whereupon, at 11:41 a.m., the Subcommittee was adjourned.]

Appendix: Answers to Post-Hearing Questions

Responses by Dr. Stephen Streiffer

Question for the Record to:

Dr. Stephen Streiffer

Deputy Laboratory Director for Science and Technology

Argonne National Laboratory

House Committee on Science, Space, and Technology

Subcommittee on Investigations and Oversight

COVID-19 Variants and Evolving Research Needs

May 12, 2021

Submitted by: Representative Sean Casten (IL-06)

What distinguishes DOE's role from that of other agencies in conducting research on COVID -19 variants?

The DOE and its 17 National Laboratories are distinguished by unique capabilities that are applicable to the threats posed by COVID-19, that are leveraged directly from core missions in fundamental research (including its scientific user facilities), applied energy, and national security, and that complement the role and expertise of other agencies. This includes a significant portfolio in biological and environmental research and bioenergy production, underscoring the concept of the energy-environment-climate nexus. More specifically, DOE's state-of-the-art user facilities and capabilities in advanced computing and artificial intelligence (AI), genomics, structural and molecular biology and biotechnology, systems modeling and decision analysis, and advanced manufacturing, among others, built up to serve the core missions, have been directly utilized by DOE national laboratories to pivot almost instantaneously to take on certain roles in the fight against COVID-19. Expertise in all of these domain science areas coupled with the DOE's nuclear security mission also leads directly to strengths in biosecurity and bioinformatics. Additionally, laboratory stewardship of DOE user facilities results in national laboratory scientists often being the strongest and most knowledgeable in applying those facilities to emerging research challenges, such as the COVID-19 pandemic.

This overarching framework has long served as the basis for strong cooperation between DOE and other federal agencies, including the National Institutes of Health (NIH), Department of Homeland Security (DHS), and Department of Defense (DoD). An example of this is that DOE is the steward of the x-ray light sources on behalf of the entire science and technology community. NIH has partnered with DOE by providing substantial NIH investment in both experimental capabilities (both capital and operations support for structural biology beamlines) at the light sources as well as research support for the structural biology community that uses those capabilities, hand-in-glove with DOE support for development and global operation of the facilities. A second example is the long-term development of extremely advanced epidemiological models at several national laboratories in cooperation with NIH and DoD, using DOE's world-leading expertise in computational science and high-performance computing, that have been rapidly adapted to COVID-19.

Taken together, DOE and its laboratories maintain as part of their on-going mission the cyber infrastructure, computational platforms, and next-generation experimental research capabilities within a single portal allowing distributed networks of scientists to work together on national emergency challenges such as COVID-19 variants. This set of platforms supports understanding the structure and function of biological systems such as SARS-CoV-2 and its variants, effectively integrating knowledge from distributed datasets, individual process components, and individual component models in an AI/machine learning-enabled, open access environment. DOE develops and maintains capabilities at user facilities that allow characterization and response to biological threats, and develops advanced instrumentation to address these research challenges. No other agency fills this role in the specific areas discussed for DOE.

Chapter 2

COVID-19 Variants: Vaccines, Diagnostics, and Therapeutics*

Amanda K. Sarata, Agata Bodie and Kavya Sekar

Introduction

As SARS-CoV-2, the virus that causes COVID-19, has spread widely over time, a number of new variants have been identified globally. According to the Centers for Disease Control and Prevention (CDC), "a new virus variant has one or more mutations that differentiate it from the wild-type or predominant virus variants already circulating among the general population." Genetic variation in circulating viruses is expected, especially with RNA viruses like SARS-CoV-2, which have high rates of mutation generally. When a virus infects its host, it uses the host cell machinery to replicate itself. This replication process is error prone and offers chances to introduce changes to the virus's genetic code. Many of these changes are inconsequential, but a few improve the fitness of the virus, providing a selective advantage and establishing new strains of the virus, which would be expected to increase in prevalence over time. Although they may occur in any part of the viral genome, changes in the genetic code for the virus part that locks onto the host cell, known as the "spike protein," have been noted in certain SARS-CoV-2 variants. These changes appear to strengthen viral attachment to the host cell, which can result in more efficient viral transmission (increased

* This is an edited, reformatted and augmented version of Congressional Research Service Publication No. IF11789, updated October 29, 2021.

In: A Closer Look at the COVID-19 Variants
Editor: Richard D. Hylton
ISBN: 979-8-88697-170-5

infectiousness). This type of change does not have to correlate with a change in the clinical severity of infection (virulence), although it may.

Currently, the Delta variant is the predominant variant strain circulating in the United States, according to CDC data. Federal agencies are actively monitoring other variants of possible concern. Certain variants, both existing and potential, may pose possible challenges to the effectiveness of existing countermeasures—vaccines, diagnostics, and therapeutics—and the development of new ones. Efforts have increased nationally to track the emergence and spread of new variants, primarily through increasing genomic and other surveillance.

Given these concerns, Congress, in the American Rescue Plan Act of 2021 (ARPA; P.L. 117-2) appropriated $1.75 billion to CDC specifically for SARS-CoV-2 genomic sequencing and surveillance; other funding in the bill, such as for data modernization and forecasting, may also aid with variant tracking, as well as with coordination of such efforts at the federal level. CDC has also used appropriations from several prior coronavirus supplemental appropriations acts to expand such efforts. P.L. 117-2 further provided funding to the Food and Drug Administration (FDA) to support, among other things, the continued evaluation of COVID-19 countermeasures, including with respect to emerging variants.

Tracking and Studying Variants

Identifying, tracking, and studying virus variants primarily relies on two public health functions: (1) genomic surveillance, based on sequencing, and (2) genomic epidemiology, which studies the health effects associated with different variants. Increasing SARS-CoV-2 genomic sequencing to facilitate surveillance in the United States has posed a challenge. Though genomic sequencing capacity exists in the academic and private laboratory sector, these sectors have not been well connected to the public health or health care sectors to readily enable large-scale and coordinated laboratory sample and data sharing for a nationwide virus sequencing effort. CDC has funded efforts and partnerships to increase genomic sequencing and surveillance since fall 2020, including through collecting specimens for sequencing, and by partnering with academic, commercial, and public health laboratories. CDC has also awarded grants to state, local, territorial, and tribal (SLTT) public health agencies to increase their capacity for genomic surveillance. Genome sequences collected through surveillance and other sequencing efforts are shared to public repositories, such as GenBank or GISAID (global initiative on sharing avian influenza data). These efforts have boosted U.S. SARS-CoV-2 sequencing by CDC and SLTT labs from about 3,000 sequences per week in early 2021 to a range of 40,000-90,000 sequences per week in September and October.

Boosting genomic epidemiology poses another challenge. Genomic epidemiology can answer questions such as whether certain variants are associated with more severe health outcomes or reduced effectiveness of medical countermeasures, and enable the use of genomic data in outbreak response. Such efforts involve linking genomic surveillance data with other types of health data, such as on patient characteristics, outcomes, or vaccination status. In the United States, siloed health data systems, as well as other legal and institutional barriers, inhibit the data integration that would enable more robust and real-time genomic epidemiology. In addition, SLTT public health agencies have varying capacity for genomic surveillance and epidemiology for a number of reasons, including a lack of technology and trained personnel with bioinformatics expertise, among others. This sector is also already strained by other aspects of the COVID-19 response. The Biden Administration has allocated the ARPA genomic surveillance funds in an effort to address these issues: $1 billion for CDC and SLTT health agencies to expand sequencing, $400 million for new Centers of Excellence in Genomic Epidemiology, and $300 million for a National Bioinformatics Infrastructure. Even with new funding, it may take time to build the infrastructure for robust nationwide genomic surveillance and epidemiology, and some legal and institutional barriers may remain.

Variants and Vaccines

The vaccines available thus far are designed to elicit a protective immune response to the SARS-CoV-2 spike protein. SARS-CoV-2 variants with mutations in the spike protein raise concerns that available vaccines may provide reduced protection. Data indicate that vaccines continue to provide strong protection against severe COVID-19 and death in the United States, including against currently circulating variants. To ensure that vaccines continue to provide robust protection against COVID-19, including against emerging variants, FDA has authorized, and CDC has endorsed, booster doses of the available vaccines, including heterologous boosters (i.e., a mix-and-match approach). As new variants emerge, vaccine dosing recommendations may be modified further.

Any changes to the currently approved or authorized vaccines or vaccine regimens must be reviewed and approved by FDA, as explained in the Emergency Use Authorization [EUA] for Vaccines to Prevent COVID-19 guidance. FDA does not expect vaccine developers to conduct the same large clinical trials that were required for initial EUA issuance. Instead, the effectiveness of a modified COVID-19 vaccine may be demonstrated through immunogenicity studies comparing the immune response induced by the modified vaccine against the SARS-CoV-2 variant(s) with the immune response induced by the EUA- authorized vaccine against the SARS-CoV-2 virus upon which the vaccine was originally based. FDA guidance provides recommendations for conducting studies assessing the effectiveness of a modified COVID-19 vaccine as part of the primary vaccine series and as a booster dose.

Variants and Diagnostics

The performance of COVID-19 tests, including molecular, antigen, and serology tests, may be affected by the emergence of new variants. FDA released guidance in February 2021—Policy for Evaluating Impact of Viral Mutations on COVID-19 Tests—to provide test developers with recommendations for monitoring the impact of variants on their tests' performance and considerations for test design that can mitigate the impact of variants.

Molecular tests, such as polymerase chain reaction (PCR) tests, identify the virus by detecting specific pieces of the viral genome, and have generally been developed using the same reference sequence. If a test's viral targets are altered in a variant, then the diagnostic may not detect them, generating a false negative result. This performance issue may be mitigated through the use of multiple targets in a molecular test; most EUA-authorized PCR tests do have multiple targets, often in different parts of the viral genome. Separately, antigen and serology test performance may be affected if a viral genetic mutation affects the eventual structure of viral proteins (e.g., antigens) that are targeted by, or used as components in, these tests. These changes may also lead to false negative results.

FDA has been "routinely monitoring publicly available databases and has coordinated efforts to evaluate the impact of new virus variants on tests that have received … EUA."

FDA used reports in the peer-reviewed literature on variants of clinical significance, as well as identification of mutations appearing with increasing frequency in public sequence repositories, to identify potential viral mutations or variants of concern. Test components are routinely compared against these mutations to determine the effect, if any, on test performance. FDA released a safety alert for clinical laboratory staff and health care providers in early January 2021 based on this work to alert the community about potential impacts of variants on specific EUA tests. The agency has continued to provide updates on affected tests to the diagnostics community since this time.

In September 2021, FDA issued notice of revisions to the EUAs of certain molecular, antigen, and serological tests, adding new conditions of authorization that must be met by test developers to account for new and emerging variants. Specifically, the conditions include updated labelling requirements to clarify that a test's performance is reflective of the variants circulating at the time of its clinical evaluation. In addition, developers must "evaluate the impact of SARS-CoV-2 viral mutations on your product's performance" on an ongoing basis.

Variants and Therapeutics

Several therapeutics are available for the treatment of COVID-19, and they differ with respect to their intended use (e.g., treatment of mild to moderate or severe disease) and mechanism of action (e.g., whether they target the virus itself or the body's inflammatory response). For example, FDA has granted EUA to several monoclonal antibody (mAb) products, which are intended for the treatment of mild to moderate COVID-19 in patients who are at high risk for progressing to severe disease.

The emergence of SARS-CoV-2 variants has raised concern about the effectiveness of existing therapeutics, particularly mAb products, which are designed to bind to the spike protein that allows the virus to infect the host cell in order to stop infection. In April 2021, FDA revoked the EUA for the mAb bamlanivimab, citing a "sustained increase of SARS-CoV-2 viral variants that are resistant to [it] alone resulting in the increased risk for treatment failure." The EUAs for other mAb products remain in effect (e.g., bamlanivimab and etesevimab, when administered together). FDA has further modified EUAs for authorized mAb products to require as a condition of authorization that, among other things, sponsors establish a process for monitoring genomic databases for the emergence of global variants of SARS-CoV-2 and, if requested by

FDA, provide an assessment of the authorized products' activity against "any global SARS-CoV-2 variant(s) of interest." Notably, the conditions of authorization for one mAb product (bamlanivimab and etesevimab) limit its use to those states, territories, and U.S. jurisdictions in which the combined frequency of variants resistant to it is 5% or less, as determined by FDA based on CDC data. FDA has provided recommendations for design of mAb development programs and considerations for emerging variants in guidance *(Development of Monoclonal Antibody Products Targeting SARS-CoV-2, Including Addressing the Impact of Emerging Variants, During the COVID-19 Public Health Emergency).*

Chapter 3

SARS-CoV-2 Variant Classifications and Definitions*

Centers for Disease Control and Prevention

Viruses like SARS-CoV-2 continuously evolve as changes in the genetic code (caused by genetic mutations or viral recombination) occur during replication of the genome. A lineage is a genetically closely related group of virus variants derived from a common ancestor. A variant has one or more mutations that differentiate it from other variants of the SARS- CoV-2 viruses. A recombinant is a variant created by the combination of genetic material from two different variants. As expected, multiple variants of SARS-CoV-2 have been documented in the United States and globally throughout this pandemic. To inform local outbreak investigations and understand national trends, scientists compare genetic differences between viruses to identify variants (including recombinants) and how they are related to each other.

Key Definitions

- Mutation: A mutation refers to a single change in a virus's genome (genetic code). Mutations happen frequently, but only sometimes change the characteristics of the virus.
- Recombinant: A process in which the genomes of two SARS-CoV-2 variants (that have infected a person at the same time) combine during

---

* This is an edited, reformatted and augmented version of CDC - Centers for Disease Control and Prevention Publication, updated April 26, 2022.

In: A Closer Look at the COVID-19 Variants
Editor: Richard D. Hylton
ISBN: 979-8-88697-170-5

the viral replication process to form a new variant that is different from both parent lineages.

- Lineage: A lineage is a group of closely related viruses with a common ancestor. SARS-CoV-2 has many lineages; all cause COVID-19.
- Variant: A variant is a viral genome (genetic code) that may contain one or more mutations. In some cases, a group of variants with similar genetic changes, such as a lineage or group of lineages, may be designated by public health organizations as a Variant Being Monitored (VBM) Variant of Concern (VOC) or a Variant of Interest (VOI) due to shared attributes and characteristics that may require public health action.

Key Points

- Genetic lineages of SARS-CoV-2 have been emerging and circulating around the world since the beginning of the COVID-19 pandemic.
- SARS-CoV-2 genetic lineages in the United States are routinely monitored through epidemiological investigations, virus genetic sequence-based surveillance, and laboratory studies.
- On November 30, 2021, the U.S. government SARS-CoV-2 Interagency Group (SIG) classifed Omicron as a Variant of Concern (VOC). This classifcation was based on the following:
  - Detection of cases attributed to Omicron in multiple countries, including among those without travel history.
  - Transmission and replacement of the Delta variant in South Africa.
  - The number and locations of substitutions in the spike protein.
  - Available data for other variants with fewer substitutions in the spike protein that indicate a reduction in neutralization by sera from vaccinated or convalescent individuals.
  - Available data for other variants with fewer substitutions in the spike protein that indicate reduced susceptibility to certain monoclonal antibody treatments.
- On April 14, 2022 the U.S government SARS-CoV-2 Interagency Group (SIG) downgraded Delta from a Variant of Concern to a

Variant Being Monitored. This new classification was based on the following:

- Significant and sustained reduction in its national and regional proportions over time.
- Evidence suggesting that Delta does not currently pose a significant risk to public health in the United States.

The SIG Variant classification scheme defines four classes of SARS-CoV-2 variants:

1. *Variant Being Monitored (VBM)*
   - Alpha (B.1.1.7 and Q lineages)
   - Beta (B.1.351 and descendent lineages)
   - Gamma (P.1 and descendent lineages)
   - Delta (B.1.617.2 and AY lineages)
   - Epsilon (B.1.427 and B.1.429)
   - Eta (B.1.525)
   - Iota (B.1.526)
   - Kappa (B.1.617.1) 1.617.3
   - Mu (B.1.621, B.1.621.1)
   - Zeta (P.2)
2. *Variant of Interest (VOI)*
3. *Variant of Concern (VOC)*
   - Omicron (B.1.1.529, BA.1, BA.1.1, BA.2, BA.3, BA.4 and BA.5 lineages)
4. *Variant of High Consequence (VOHC)*

To date, no variants of high consequence have been identified in the United States.

Vaccines approved and authorized for use in the United States are effective against the predominant variant circulating in the United States and effective therapeutics are available. CDC continues to monitor all variants circulating within the United States.

How Variants Are Classified

The U.S. Department of Health and Human Services (HHS) established a SARS-CoV-2 Interagency Group (SIG) to enhance coordination among CDC,

National Institutes of Health (NIH), Food and Drug Administration (FDA), Biomedical Advanced Research and Development Authority (BARDA), and Department of Defense (DoD). This interagency group is focused on the rapid characterization of emerging variants and actively monitors their potential impact on critical SARS-CoV-2 countermeasures, including vaccines, therapeutics, and diagnostics.

The SIG meets regularly to evaluate the risk posed by SARS-CoV-2 variants circulating in the United States and to make recommendations about the classification of variants. This evaluation is undertaken by a group of subject matter experts who assess available data, including variant proportions at the national and regional levels and the potential or known impact of the constellation of mutations on the effectiveness of medical countermeasures, severity of disease, and ability to spread from person to person. Given the continuous evolution of SARS-CoV-2 and our understanding of the impact of variants on public health, variants may be reclassified based on their attributes and prevalence in the United States.

- Variants Being Monitored (VBM)
- Variant of Interest (VOI)
- Variant of Concern (VOC)
- Variant of High Consequence (VOHC)

Each variant classification includes the possible attributes of lower classes (for example, VOC includes the possible attributes of VOI); variant status might escalate or deescalate based on emerging scientific evidence. The World Health Organization (WHO) also classifies variant viruses as variants of concern and variants of interest; U.S. classifications may differ from those of WHO because the impact of variants may differ by location. To assist with public discussions of variants, WHO proposed using labels consisting of the Greek alphabet (for example, alpha, beta, gamma) as a practical way to discuss variants for non-scientific audiences.

Variants Being Monitored (VBM)

CDC monitors all variants circulating in the United States. Variants designated as VBM include those where data indicates there is a potential or clear impact on approved or authorized medical countermeasures or that have been associated with more severe disease or increased transmission but are no longer detected, or are circulating at very low levels, in the United States. These variants do not pose a significant and imminent risk to public health in the United States.

A Variant of Interest or a Variant of Concern may be downgraded to this list after a significant and sustained reduction in its national and regional proportions over time, or other evidence indicates that a variant does not pose significant risk to public health in the United States.

These variants continue to be closely monitored to identify changes in their proportions and new data are continually being analyzed. If the data indicate that a VBM warrants more concern, the classification will be changed based on the SIG assessment of the attributes of the variant and the risk to public health in the United States.

WHO Label	**Pango Lineage**	**Date of Designation**		
Alpha	B.1.1.7 and Q lineages	VOC: December 29, 2020		VBM: September 21, 2021
Beta	B.1.351 and descendent lineages	VOC: December 29, 2020		VBM: September 21, 2021
Gamma	P.1and descendent lineages	VOC: December 29, 2020		VBM: September 21, 2021
Delta	B.1.617.2 and AY lineages	VOC: June 15, 2021		VBM: April 14, 2022
Epsilon	B.1.427 B.1.429	VOC: March 19, 2021	VOI: February 26, 2021 VOI: June 29, 2021	VBM: September 21, 2021
Eta	B.1.525		VOI: February 26, 2021	VBM: September 21, 2021
Iota	B.1.526		VOI: February 26, 2021	VBM: September 21, 2021
Kappa	B.1.617.1		VOI: May 7, 2021	VBM: September 21, 2021
N/A	B.1.617.3		VOI: May 7, 2021	VBM: September 21, 2021

(Continued)

WHO Label	Pango Lineage	Date of Designation		
Zeta	P.2		VOI: February 26, 2021	VBM: September 21, 2021
Mu	B.1.621 B.1.621.1			VBM: September 21, 2021

Variant of Interest (VOI)

A variant with specific genetic markers that have been associated with changes to receptor binding, reduced neutralization by antibodies generated against previous infection or vaccination, reduced efficacy of treatments, potential diagnostic impact, or predicted increase in transmissibility or disease severity.

Possible attributes of a Variant of Interest:

- Specific genetic markers that are predicted to affect transmission, diagnostics, therapeutics, or immune escape.
- Evidence that it is the cause of an increased proportion of cases or unique outbreak clusters.
- Limited prevalence or expansion in the US or in other countries.

A Variant of Interest might require one or more appropriate public health actions, including enhanced sequence surveillance, enhanced laboratory characterization, or epidemiological investigations to assess how easily the virus spreads to others, the severity of disease, the efficacy of therapeutics and whether currently approved or authorized vaccines offer protection.

Currently, no SARS-CoV-2 variants are designated as VOI.

Variant of Concern (VOC)

A variant for which there is evidence of an increase in transmissibility, more severe disease (for example, increased hospitalizations or deaths), significant reduction in neutralization by antibodies generated during previous infection or vaccination, reduced effectiveness of treatments or vaccines, or diagnostic detection failures.

Possible attributes of a variant of concern in addition to the possible attributes of a variant of interest:

- Evidence of impact on diagnostics, treatments, or vaccines
  - Widespread interference with diagnostic test targets
  - Evidence of substantially decreased susceptibility to one or more class of therapies
  - Evidence of significantly decreased neutralization by antibodies generated during previous infection or vaccination
  - Evidence of reduced vaccine-induced protection from severe disease
- Evidence of increased transmissibility
- Evidence of increased disease severity

Variants of concern might require one or more appropriate public health actions, such as notification to WHO under the International Health Regulations, reporting to CDC, local or regional efforts to control spread, increased testing, or research to determine the effectiveness of vaccines and treatments against the variant. Based on the characteristics of the variant, additional considerations may include the development of new diagnostics or the modification of vaccines or treatments.

Current variants of concern in the United States that are being closely monitored and characterized are listed below. This table will be updated when a new variant of concern is identified.

Footnotes for Variants of Concern

(*) = detected in some sequences but not all.

a. Phylogenetic Assignment of Named Global Outbreak (PANGO) Lineages is software tool developed by members of the Rambaut Lab. The associated web application was developed by the Centre for Genomic Pathogen Surveillance in South Cambridgeshire and is intended to implement the dynamic nomenclature of SARS-CoV-2 lineages, known as the PANGO nomenclature.
b. Nextstrain, a collaboration between researchers in Seattle, USA and Basel, Switzerland, provides open-source tools for visualizing the

genetics of outbreaks. The goal is to support public health surveillance by facilitating understanding of the spread and evolution of pathogens.

Variant of High Consequence (VOHC)

A VOHC has clear evidence that prevention measures or medical countermeasures (MCMs) have significantly reduced effectiveness relative to previously circulating variants.

Possible attributes of a variant of high consequence, in addition to the possible attributes of a variant of concern:

- Impact on MCMs
  - Demonstrated failure of diagnostic test targets
  - Evidence to suggest a significant reduction in vaccine effectiveness, a disproportionately high number of infections in vaccinated persons, or very low vaccine-induced protection against severe disease
  - Significantly reduced susceptibility to multiple EUA or approved therapeutics
  - More severe clinical disease and increased hospitalizations

A variant of high consequence would require notification to WHO under the International Health Regulations, reporting to CDC, an announcement of strategies to prevent or contain transmission, and recommendations to update treatments and vaccines.

Currently, no SARS-CoV-2 variants are designated as VOHC.

Characteristics of Selected SARS-CoV-2 Variants

- *WHO Label:* Omicron
- *Pango Lineage:* B.1.1.529, BA.1, BA.1.1, BA.2, BA.3, BA.4 and BA.5 lineages (Pango lineage)[a]
- *Spike Protein Substitutions:* A67V, del69-70, T95I, del142-144, Y145D, del211, L212I, ins214EPE, G339D, S371L, S373P, S375F,

K417N, N440K, G446S, S477N, T478K, E484A, Q493R, G496S, Q498R, N501Y, Y505H, T547K, D614G, H655Y, N679K, P681H, N764K, D796Y, N856K, Q954H, N969K, L981F

- *Nextstrain clade* (Nextstrain)[b]: 21K
- *First Identified:* South Africa
- *Attributes:*
  - Potential increased transmissibility
  - Potential reduction in neutralization by some EUA monoclonal antibody treatments
  - Potential reduction in neutralization by post-vaccination sera

Substitutions of Concern for SARS-CoV-2 Monoclonal Antibody Therapies

In the United States, there are three anti-SARS-CoV-2 monoclonal antibody treatments with FDA Emergency Use Authorization (EUA) for the treatment of COVID-19: bamlanivimab plus etesevimab, casirivimab plus imdevimab, and sotrovimab.

CDC's national genomic surveillance program identifies new and emerging SARS-CoV-2 variants to determine implications for COVID-19 diagnostics, treatments, or vaccines approved or authorized for use in the United States. Sequences with similar genetic changes are grouped into lineages, and multiple lineages can have the same substitutions. For example, the E484K substitution is found in lineages B.1.351, P.1, B.1.526, and many others. Genomic surveillance efforts provide the capability to detect viruses that have reduced susceptibility to treatments more quickly.

Reduced susceptibility of SARS-CoV-2 to sotrovimab or the combination of casirivimab and imdevimab has not been reported. In laboratory studies, SARS-CoV-2 variants that contain certain substitutions in the spike protein have reduced susceptibility to the combination of bamlanivimab and etesevimab. Clinicians seeking advice on the use of monoclonal antibody products authorized for emergency use in the United States for the treatment and prevention of SARS-CoV-2 should consult the NIH COVID-19 Treatment Guidelines.

Given the predominance of the Delta variant in the United States, it is important to note that the vast majority of Delta variant lineages are sensitive to the combination of bamlanivimab and etesevimab. Although Delta variants contain the L452R substitution, the combination of the L452R and T478K substitutions found in most Delta variants results in no change in the susceptibility to the combination of bamlanivimab and etesevimab, as noted in the FDA Fact Sheet for Health Care Providers.

The proportion data below show the national and regional unweighted proportions of SARS-CoV-2 that contain the following individual or combinations of spike protein substitutions that reduce susceptibility to the combination of bamlanivimab and etesevimab that are listed in the FDA Fact Sheet for Health Care Providers for EUA of Bamlanivimab and Etesevimab. As new data become available, additional substitutions may be added below. The national and regional proportions provided below will be updated weekly.

- L452R
- E484K
- L452R and E484Q
- K417N, E484K, and N501Y
- K417T, E484K, and N501Y
- K417N, L452R, and T478K
- R346K, E484K, and N501Y

Unweighted Proportions of SARS-CoV-2 Substitutions of Therapeutic Concern

1. L452R Spike Protein Substitution National Proportion[a]: 93.8%
    - Regional Proportions[b]
        - Region 1: 98.3%
        - Region 2: 94.4%
        - Region 3: 97.9%
        - Region 4: 94.3%
        - Region 5: 92.0%
        - Region 6: 91.7%
        - Region 7: 93.9%
        - Region 8: 96.3%
        - Region 9: 91.1%
        - Region 10: 96.3%

- Common Pango Lineages with Spike Protein Substitutions[c]
  - B.1.617.2 (Delta)
  - AY.4 (Delta)
  - AY.3 (Delta)
  - AY.12 (Delta)
  - AY.3.1 (Delta)
  - AY.14 (Delta)
  - AY.20 (Delta)
  - AY.25 (Delta)

2. E484K Spike Protein Substitution National Proportion[a]: 0.3%
   - Regional Proportions[b]
     - Region 1: 0.5%
     - Region 2: 0.4%
     - Region 3: 0.2%
     - Region 4: 0.2%
     - Region 5: 0.2%
     - Region 6: 0.2%
     - Region 7: 0.1%
     - Region 8: 0.1%
     - Region 9: 0.2%
     - Region 10: 0.4%
   - Common Pango Lineages with Spike Protein Substitutions[c]
     - B.1.621(Mu)
     - P.1 (Gamma)
     - B.1.621.1 (Mu)
     - P.1.7 (Gamma)
     - P.1.4 (Gamma)
     - P.1.10 (Gamma)
     - B.1.617.2 (Delta)
     - B.1.626
     - B.1.632

3. K417N, E484K, N501Y Spike Protein Substitution National Proportion[a]: ≤0.3%
   - Regional Proportions[b]
     - Region 1: 0.0%

  - Region 2: 0.0%
  - Region 3: 0.0%
  - Region 4: 0.0%
  - Region 5: 0.0%
  - Region 6: 0.0%
  - Region 7: 0.0%
  - Region 8: 0.0%
  - Region 9: 0.0%
  - Region 10: 0.1%
- Common Pango Lineages with Spike Protein Substitutions[c]
  - B.1.621 (Mu)
  - B.1.351 (Beta)

4. K417T, E484K, N501Y Spike Protein Substitution National Proportion[a]: 0.1%
   - Regional Proportions[b]
     - Region 1: 0.2%
     - Region 2: 0.0%
     - Region 3: 0.1%
     - Region 4: 0.1%
     - Region 5: 0.1%
     - Region 6: 0.2%
     - Region 7: 0.1%
     - Region 8: 0.0%
     - Region 9: 0.1%
     - Region 10: 0.1%
   - Common Pango Lineages with Spike Protein Substitutions[c]
     - P.1 (Gamma)
     - P.1.10 (Gamma)
     - P.1.2 (Gamma)
     - P.1.4 (Gamma)
     - P.1.7 (Gamma)

5. L452R, E484Q Spike Protein Substitution National Proportion[a]: 0.2%
   - Regional Proportions[b]
     - Region 1: 0.2%

  - Region 2: 0.2%
  - Region 3: 0.1%
  - Region 4: 0.1%
  - Region 5: 0.1%
  - Region 6: 0.3%
  - Region 7: 0.0%
  - Region 8: 0.1%
  - Region 9: 0.2%
  - Region 10: 0.1%
- Common Pango Lineages with Spike Protein Substitutions[c]
  - B.1.617.2 (Delta)
  - AY.4 (Delta)
  - AY.7.2 (Delta)
  - AY.25 (Delta)
  - AY.12 (Delta)
  - B.1.617.1 (Kappa)
  - AY.3 (Delta)
  - AY.20 (Delta)

6. K417N, L452R, T478K Spike Protein Substitution National Proportion[a]: 0.3%
   - Regional Proportions[b]
     - Region 1: 0.1%
     - Region 2: 0.3%
     - Region 3: 0.1%
     - Region 4: 0.1%
     - Region 5: 0.1%
     - Region 6: 0.0%
     - Region 7: 0.0%
     - Region 8: 0.2%
     - Region 9: 1.0%
     - Region 10: 0.3%
   - Common Pango Lineages with Spike Protein Substitutions[c]
     - AY.2 (Delta)
     - AY.1 (Delta)
     - B.1.617.2 (Delta)
     - AY.25 (Delta)

7. R346K, E484K, N501Y Spike Protein Substitution National Proportion[a]: 0.1%
   - Regional Proportions[b]
     - Region 1: 0.2%
     - Region 2: 0.3%
     - Region 3: 0.1%
     - Region 4: 0.1%
     - Region 5: 0.1%
     - Region 6: 0.1%
     - Region 7: 0.0%
     - Region 8: 0.1%
     - Region 9: 0.0%
     - Region 10: 0.3%
   - Common Pango Lineages with Spike Protein Substitutions[c]
     - B.1.621.(Mu)
     - B.1.621.1.(Mu)

Footnotes for Unweighted Proportions of SARS-CoV-2 Substitutions of Therapeutic Concern

a. The unweighted proportion of SARS-CoV-2 circulating in the United States that contain the designated substitution, based on > 60,000 sequences collected through CDC's national genomic surveillance during the two-week period ending August 28, 2021.
b. The unweighted regional proportion of SARS-CoV-2 circulating in each HHS region that contain the designated substitution, based on > 60,000 sequences collected through CDC's national genomic surveillance during the two-week period ending August 28, 2021.
c. The lineages listed are the most common lineages within CDC's national genomic surveillance with these substitutions, but this list is not intended to be a complete list of the lineages that contain the spike protein substitutions.

References

[1] Zhou, B., Thao, T. T. N., Hoffmann, D., Taddeo, A., Ebert, N., Labroussaa, F., Pohlmann, A., King, J., Steiner, S., Kelly, J. N., Portmann, J., Halwe, N. J., Ulrich, L., Trüeb, B. S., Fan, X., Hoffmann, B., Wang, L., Thomann, L., Lin, X., … Beer, M. (2021). SARS-CoV-2 spike D614G change enhances replication and transmission. *Nature* (2021). https://doi.org/10.1038/s41586-021-03361-1.

[2] Volz, E., Hill, V., McCrone, J. T., Price, A., Jorgensen, D., O'Toole, Á., Southgate, J., Johnson, R., Jackson, B., Nascimento, F. F., Rey, S. M., Nicholls, S. M., Colquhoun, R. M., da Silva Filipe, A., Shepherd, J., Pascall, D. J., Shah, R., Jesudason, N., Li, K., … Neaverson, A. S. (2021). Evaluating the effects of SARS-CoV-2 spike mutation D614G on transmissibility and pathogenicity. *Cell* 2021; 184(64-75). doi: https://doi.org/10.1016/j.cell.2020.11.020.

[3] Korber, B., Fischer, W. M., Gnanakaran, S., Yoon, H., Theiler, J., Abfalterer, W., Hengartner, N., Giorgi, E. E., Bhattacharya, T., Foley, B., Hastie, K. M., Parker, M. D., Partridge, D. G., Evans, C. M., Freeman, T. M., de Silva, T. I., McDanal, C., Perez, L. G., Tang, H., … Wyles, M. D. (2020). Tracking changes in SARS-CoV-2 spike: Evidence that D614G increases infectivity of the COVID-19 virus. *Cell* 2021; 182(812-7) doi: https://doi.org/10.1016/ j.cell.2020.06.043.

[4] Yurkovetskiy, L., Wang, X., Pascal, K. E., Tomkins-Tinch, C., Nyalile, T., Wang, Y., Baum, A., Diehl, W. E., Dauphin, A., Carbone, C., Veinotte, K., Egri, S., Schaffner, S., Lemieux, J. E., Munro, J., Rafique, A., Barve, A., Sabeti, P. C., Kyratsous, C. A., … Luban, J. (2020). Structural and functional analysis of the D614G SARS-CoV-2 spike protein variant. *Cell* 2020; 183(3): 739-751. doi: https://doi.org/ 10.1016/j.cell.2020.09.032.

[5] * Davies, N. G., Abbott, S., Barnard, R. C., Jarvis, C. I., Kucharski, A. J., Munday, J. D., Pearson, C. A. B., Russell, T. W., Tully, D. C., Washburne, A. D., Wenseleers, T., Gimma, A., Waites, W., Wong, K. L. M., van Zandvoort, K., Silverman, J. D., CMMID COVID-19 Working Group, COVID-19 Genomics UK (COG-UK) Consortium, Diaz-Ordaz, K., … Edmunds, W. J. (2021). Estimated transmissibility and impact of SARS-CoV-2 lineage B.1.1.7 in England. *MedRXiv* 2021. doi: https://doi.org/10.1101/2020.12.24.20248822.

[6] Horby P, Huntley C, Davies N et al. NERVTAG note on B.1.1.7 severity. New & emerging threats advisory group, Jan. 21, 2021. Retrieved from *NERVTAG Note on Variant Severity.*

[7] FDA. *Fact Sheet For Health Care Providers Emergency Use Authorization (Eua) Of Bamlanivimab And Etesevimab 02092021.* fda.gov.

[8] * Wang, P., Nair, M. S., Liu, L., Iketani, S., Luo, Y., Guo, Y., Wang, M., Yu, J., Zhang, B., Kwong, P. D., Graham, B. S., Mascola, J. R., Chang, J. Y., Yin, M. T., Sobieszczyk, M., Kyratsous, C. A., Shapiro, L., Sheng, Z., Huang, Y., & Ho, D. D. (2021). Antibody Resistance of SARS-CoV-2 Variants B.1.351 and B.1.1.7. *BioXRiv 2021.* doi: https://doi.org/ 10.1101/2021.01.25.428137.

[9] * Shen, X., Tang, H., McDanal, C., Wagh, K., Fischer, W., Theiler, J., Yoon, H., Li, D., Haynes, B. F., Sanders, K. O., Gnanakaran, S., Hengartner, N., Pajon, R., Smith, G., Glenn, G. M., Korber, B., & Montefiori, D. C. (2021). SARS-CoV-2 variant

B.1.1.7 is susceptible to neutralizing antibodies elicited by ancestral Spike vaccines. *BioRxiv 2021.* doi: https://doi.org/10.1101/2021.01.27. 428516.

[10] *Edara V V, Floyd K, Lai L, et al. Infection and mRNA-1273 vaccine antibodies neutralize SARS-CoV-2 UK variant. *MedRxiv 2021.* doi: https://doi.org/10.1101/2021.02.02.21250799.

[11] *Collier D A, DeMarco A, Ferreira I, et al. SARS-CoV-2 B.1.1.7 sensitivity to mRNA vaccine-elicited, convalescent and monoclonal antibodies. *MedRxiv* 2021. doi:https://doi.org/10.1101/2021.01.19.2 1249840.

[12] *Wu K, Werner A P, Moliva J I, et al. mRNA-1273 vaccine induces neutralizing antibodies against spike mutants from global SARS-CoV-2 variants. *BioRxiv 2021.* doi:https://doi.org/10.1101/2021.01.25.4279 48.

[13] Emary, K. R. W., Golubchik, T., Aley, P. K., Ariani, C. V., Angus, B., Bibi, S., Blane, B., Bonsall, D., Cicconi, P., Charlton, S., Clutterbuck, E. A., Collins, A. M., Cox, T., Darton, T. C., Dold, C., Douglas, A. D., Duncan, C. J. A., Ewer, K. J., Flaxman, A. L., … Pollard, A. J. (2021). Efficacy of ChAdOx1 nCoV-19 (AZD1222) Vaccine Against SARS-CoV-2 VOC 202012/01 (B.1.1.7). 2021. *The Lancet*. doi: http://dx.doi.org/10.2139/ssrn. 3779160.

[14] FACT SHEET FOR HEALTH CARE PROVIDERS EMERGENCY USE AUTHORIZATION (EUA) OF REGEN-COV (fda.gov).

[15] * Wang, P., Casner, R. G., Nair, M. S., Wang, M., Yu, J., Cerutti, G., Liu, L., Kwong, P. D., Huang, Y., Shapiro, L., & Ho, D. D. (2021). Increased resistance of SARS-CoV-2 variant P.1 to antibody neutralization. *BioRxiv* 2021. doi: https://doi. org/10.1101/2021.03.01. 433466.

[16] Pearson C A B, Russell T W, Davies N G, et al. Estimates of severity and transmissibility of novel South Africa SARS- CoV-2 variant 501Y.V2. Retrieved from: cmmid.github.io.

[17] Liu, Y., Liu, J., Xia, H., Zhang, X., Fontes-Garfias, C. R., Swanson, K. A., Cai, H., Sarkar, R., Chen, W., Cutler, M., Cooper, D., Weaver, S. C., Muik, A., Sahin, U., Jansen, K. U., Xie, X., Dormitzer, P. R., & Shi, P.-Y. (2021). Neutralizing activity of BNT162b2-elicited serum. 2021. *NEJM.* doi: 10.1056/NEJMc2102017.

[18] * Madhi, S. A., Baillie, V., Cutland, C. L., Voysey, M., Koen, A. L., Fairlie, L., Padayachee, S. D., Dheda, K., Barnabas, S. L., Bhorat, Q. E., Briner, C., Kwatra, G., Ahmed, K., Aley, P., Bhikha, S., Bhiman, J. N., Bhorat, A. E., du Plessis, J., Esmail, A., … Izu, A. (2021). Safety and effiacy of the ChAdOx1 nCoV-19 (AZD1222) Covid-19 vaccine against the B.1.351 variant in South Africa. *MedRxiv* 2021. doi: https://doi.org/10.1101/ 2021.02.10.21251247.

[19] Novavax Inc. Novavax COVID-19 vaccine demonstrates 89.3% efficacy in UK Phase 3 trial. IR Site.

[20] Johnson & Johnson. Johnson & Johnson COVID-19 vaccine authorized by U.S. FDA for emergency use. jnj.com.

[21] *Deng X, Garcia-Knight M A, Khalid M M, et al. Transmission, infectivity, and antibody neutralization of an emerging SARS-CoV-2 variant in California carrying a L452R spike protein mutation. *MedRxiv* 2021. doi: https://doi.org/10.1101/ 2021.03.07.21252647.

[22] Xie X, Liu Y, Liu J, et al. SARS-CoV-2 spike E484K mutation reduces antibody neutralisation. *The Lancet* 2021. doi: https://doi.org/10.1016/S2666-5247(21)00068-9.

[23] Garcia-Beltran, W. F., Lam, E. C., St. Denis, K., Nitido, A. D., Garcia, Z. H., Hauser, B. M., Feldman, J., Pavlovic, M. N., Gregory, D. J., Poznansky, M. C., Sigal, A., Schmidt, A. G., Iafrate, A. J., Naranbhai, V., & Balazs, A. B. (2021). Multiple SARS-CoV-2 variants escape neutralization by vaccine-induced humoral immunity. *Cell 2021*. doi: https://doi.org/10.1016/j.cell.2021.03.013.

[24] *Annavajhala M K, Mohri H, Zucker J E, at al. A Novel SARS-CoV-2 Variant of concern, B.1.526, identified in New York. *MedRxiv 2021.* doi: 1101/2021.02.23.21252259.

[25] *Yadav P D, Sapkal G N, Abraham P, et al. Neutralization of variant under investigation B.1.617 with sera of BBV152 vaccinees. *BioRxiv 2021*. doi: https://doi.org/10.1101/2021.04.23.441101.

[26] Greaney, A. J., Loes, A. N., Crawford, K. H. D., Starr, T. N., Malone, K. D., Chu, H. Y., & Bloom, J. D. (2021). Comprehensive mapping of mutations in the SARS-CoV-2 receptor- binding domain that affect recognition by polyclonal human plasma antibodies. *Cell* 2021. doi: https://doi.org/10.1016/j.chom.2021.02.003.

[27] *Edara V V, Lai L, Sahoo M K, et al. Infection and vaccine-induced neutralizing antibody responses to the SARS-CoV-2 B.1.617.1 variant. *BioRxiv* 2021. doi: https://doi.org/10.1101/2021.05.09.443299.

[28] FDA. GSK Sotrovimab Fact Sheet for HCP 05262021 (fda.gov).

[29] Allen, H., Vusirikala, A., Flannagan, J., Twohig, K. A., Zaidi, A., Chudasama, D., Lamagni, T., Groves, N., Turner, C., Rawlinson, C., Lopez-Bernal, J., Harris, R., Charlett, A., Dabrera, G., & Kall, M. (2022). Increased household transmission of COVID-19 cases associated with SARS- CoV-2 Variant of Concern B.1.617.2: a national case-control study. *Public Health England.* 2021.

**Non-peer-reviewed*

Chapter 4

Understanding Variants*

Centers for Disease Control and Prevention

The virus that causes COVID-19 is constantly changing, and new variants of the virus are expected to occur. Sometimes new variants emerge and disappear. Other times, new variants persist. Numerous variants of the virus that causes COVID-19 are being tracked in the United States and globally during this pandemic.

How Variants Work

If you think about a virus like a tree growing and branching out; each branch on the tree is slightly different than the others. By comparing the branches, scientists can label them according to the differences. These small differences, or variants, have been studied and identified since the beginning of the pandemic.

Some variations allow the virus to spread more easily or make it resistant to treatments or vaccines. Those variants must be monitored more carefully.

How Variants Change

As the virus spreads, it has new opportunities to change and may become more difficult to stop. These changes can be monitored by comparing differences in

* This is an edited, reformatted and augmented version of CDC- Centers for Disease Control and Prevention Publication, updated August 6, 2021.

In: A Closer Look at the COVID-19 Variants
Editor: Richard D. Hylton
ISBN: 979-8-88697-170-5

physical traits (such as resistance to treatment) or changes in genetic code (mutations) from one variant to another.

What We Are Doing

By studying each variant and understanding these differences, scientists can monitor, and often predict, whether a variant is more dangerous than others. Scientists can also use this information to track the spread of a variant.

Important Ways to Slow the Spread of COVID-19

- Get vaccinated and stay up to date on your COVID-19 vaccines. Find a vaccine.
- Wear a well-fitted mask to help protect yourself and others.
- Avoid crowds and poorly ventilated indoor spaces.
- Test to prevent spread to others.
- Stay 6 feet apart from others who don't live with you.
- Wash your hands often with soap and water. Use hand sanitizer if soap and water aren't available.

Chapter 5

What You Need to Know About Variants*

Centers for Disease Control and Prevention

What You Need to Know

- New variants of the virus are expected to occur.
- Slowing the spread of the virus, by protecting yourself and others can help slow the emergence of new variants.
- The Omicron variant causes more infections and spreads faster than the original SARS-CoV-2 strain of the virus that causes COVID-19.
- CDC is working with state and local public health officials to monitor the spread of all variants, including Omicron.
- Getting a vaccine reduces your risk of severe illness, hospitalization, and death from COVID-19. Staying up to date on your COVID-19 vaccines, which includes getting a booster when eligible, further improves your protection.

Variants Are Expected

Viruses constantly change through mutation and sometimes these mutations result in a new variant of the virus. Some variants emerge and disappear while others persist. New variants will continue to emerge. CDC and other public

* This is an edited, reformatted and augmented version of CDC- Centers for Disease Control and Prevention Publication, updated April 26, 2022.

In: A Closer Look at the COVID-19 Variants
Editor: Richard D. Hylton
ISBN: 979-8-88697-170-5

health organizations monitor all variants of the virus that causes COVID-19 in the United States and globally.

Scientists monitor all variants but may classify certain ones as variants being monitored variants of interest, variants of concern and variants of high consequence. Some variants spread more easily and quickly than other variants, which may lead to more cases of COVID-19. Even if a variant causes less severe disease in general, an increase in the overall number of cases could cause an increase in hospitalizations, put more strain on healthcare resources and potentially lead to more deaths.

Variants of Concern

Omicron - B.1.1.529, BA.1, BA.1.1, BA.2, BA.3, BA.4 and BA.5

- *First identified*: South Africa.
- *Spread*: Spreads more easily than other variants. CDC is working with state and local public health officials to monitor the spread of Omicron.
- *Symptoms*: Fever or chills, cough, shortness of breath or difficulty breathing, fatigue, muscle or body aches, headache, new loss of taste or smell, sore throat, congestion or runny nose, nausea or vomiting, diarrhea.
- *Severe illness and death*: Data suggest that Omicron is less severe in general. However, a surge in cases may lead to significant increases in hospitalization and death. More data are needed to fully understand the severity of illness and death associated with this variant.
- *Vaccine*: Breakthrough infections in people who are vaccinated are expected, but being up to date on recommended vaccines is effective at preventing severe illness, hospitalizations, and death. The emergence of the Omicron variant further emphasizes the importance of vaccination and boosters.
- *Treatments*: Some, but not all, monoclonal antibody treatments remain effective against Omicron. Public health agencies work with healthcare providers to ensure that effective treatments are used appropriately to treat patients.

We Have the Tools to Fight COVID-19

Vaccines

- Vaccines reduce the risk of severe illness, hospitalization, and death from COVID-19.
- People who are up to date on vaccines, including booster doses when eligible are likely to have stronger protection against COVID-19 variants, including Omicron. CDC recommends everyone eligible get vaccinated and a booster shot.

Masks

When to Wear a Mask

- Wear a well-fitting mask with the best fit, protection, and comfort for you.
- If you are in an area with a high COVID-19 Community Level and are ages 2 or older, wear a well-fitting mask indoors in public.
- If you are sick and need to be around others, or are caring for someone who has COVID-19, wear a mask.
- If you are at increased risk for severe illness, or live with or spend time with someone at higher risk, speak to your healthcare provider about wearing a mask at medium COVID-19 Community Levels.

Testing

- Tests for COVID-19 tell you if you have an infection at the time of the test. This type of test is called a "viral" test because it looks for viral infection. Antigen or Nucleic Acid Amplification Tests (NAATs) are viral tests.
  - Additional tests would be needed to determine which variant caused your infection, but these typically are not authorized for public use.
- As new variants emerge, scientists will continue to evaluate how well tests detect current infection.

- Self-tests may be used if you have COVID-19 symptoms or have been exposed or potentially exposed to an individual with COVID-19.
  - Even if you don't have symptoms and have not been exposed to an individual with COVID-19, using a self-test before gathering indoors with others can give you information about the risk of spreading the virus that causes COVID-19.

Chapter 6

Vaccinations > Variants*

Centers for Disease Control and Prevention

After experiencing a brief decline in COVID-19, the United States is once again seeing an increase in cases in most of the country. This recent increase follows a previous summer surge that was fueled by the highly contagious Delta (B.1.617.2) variant and low vaccination coverage in many communities. COVID-19 vaccines offer strong protection against serious illness and death. High vaccination coverage is proven to reduce the spread of the virus. The less a virus spreads, the less opportunity there is for new variants to emerge.

The virus that causes COVID-19 constantly changes, or mutates, producing new variants of the virus. The Delta variant continues to be the predominant strain in the United States, making up more than 99% of cases. On August 30, 2021, the World Health Organization classified the Mu (B.1.621) variant as a Variant of Interest (VOI). CDC has not designated Mu as a VOI at this time. The Mu variant reached a peak in the United States in late June 2021 and has steadily declined since then.[1] CDC continues to study and monitor all known variants and will continue to provide information when variants change classification in the United States.

Getting vaccinated is the best way to protect yourself, your family, and your community. It is also the best way to prevent new variants from emerging. A recent CDC study found that people who were not fully vaccinated had about 10 times the risk of being hospitalized with or dying

* This is an edited, reformatted and augmented version of CDC- Centers for Disease Control and Prevention Publication, Interpretive Summary for September 17, 2021.

[1] At its peak, Mu made up less than 5% of all variants circulating in the United States. Currently, Mu makes up less than 1% of all COVID-19 cases in the United States.

In: A Closer Look at the COVID-19 Variants
Editor: Richard D. Hylton
ISBN: 979-8-88697-170-5

from COVID-19 compared with people who were fully vaccinated. CDC recommends that everyone in the United States 12 years and older get vaccinated as soon as possible.

Reported Cases

The current 7-day moving average of daily new cases (146,182) increased 6.1% compared with the previous 7-day moving average (137,783). A total of 41,593,179 COVID-19 cases have been reported as of September 15, 2021.

- *Total Cases Reported*: 41,593,179
- *Current 7-Day Average*[2]: 146,182
- *Prior 7-Day Average*: 137,783
- *Change in 7-Day Average since Prior Week*: 6.1%

SARS-CoV-2 Variants

Multiple variants of the virus that causes COVID-19 are circulating globally, including within the United States. Currently, four variants are classified as a variant of concern (VOC). Nowcast estimates[3] of COVID-19 cases caused by these VOCs for the week ending September 11, 2021, are summarized here. Nationally, the combined proportion of cases attributed to Delta is estimated to be greater than 99%. The national proportions of Alpha, Beta, and Gamma are estimated to be less than 0.1%. Nowcast estimates indicate that Delta will continue to be the predominant variant circulating in all 10 U.S. Department of Health and Human Services (HHS) regions, circulating at greater than 99%. The proportions of Alpha, Beta, and Gamma are estimated to be less than or equal to 0.1% in all HHS regions.

---

[2] Historical cases are excluded from daily new cases and 7-day average calculations until they are incorporated into the dataset for the applicable date. Of 116,408 historical cases reported retroactively, 5,796 were reported in the current week and 6,516 were reported in the prior week.

[3] The median time from specimen collection to sequence data reporting is about 3 weeks. As a result, weighted estimates for the most recent few weeks may be unstable or unavailable. CDC's Nowcast is a data projection tool that helps fill this gap by generating timely estimates of variant proportions for variants that are circulating in the United States. View Nowcast estimates on CDC's COVID Data Tracker website on the Variant Proportions page.

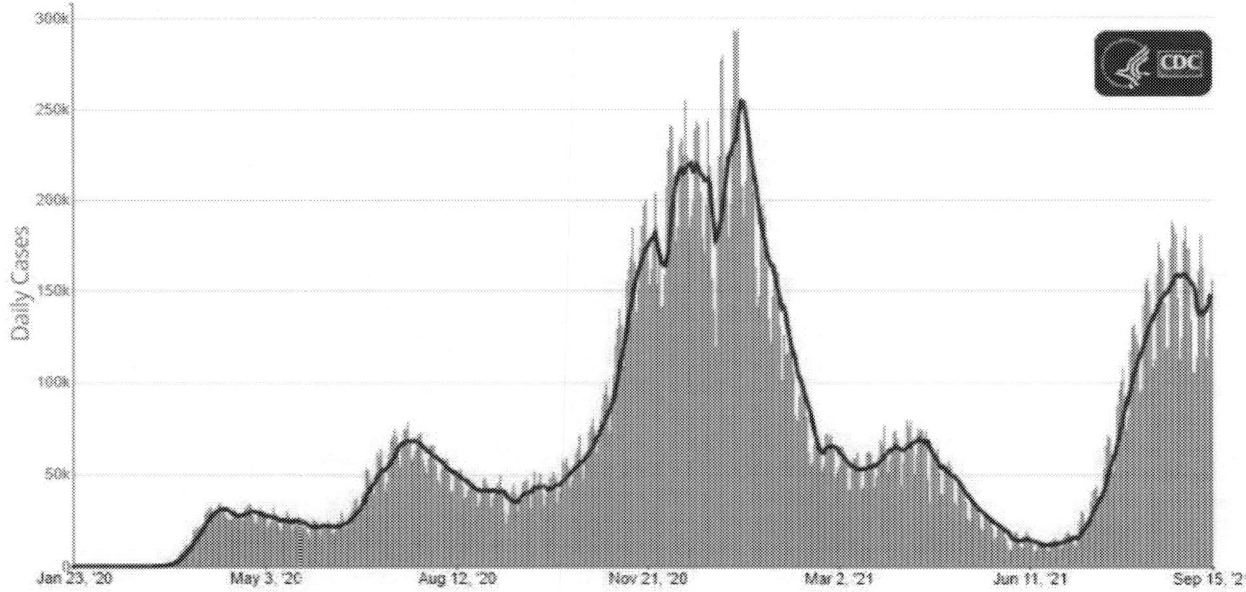

1. View

More Case Data

Daily trends in COVID-19 cases in the United States reported to CDC (red line indicates 7-day moving average).

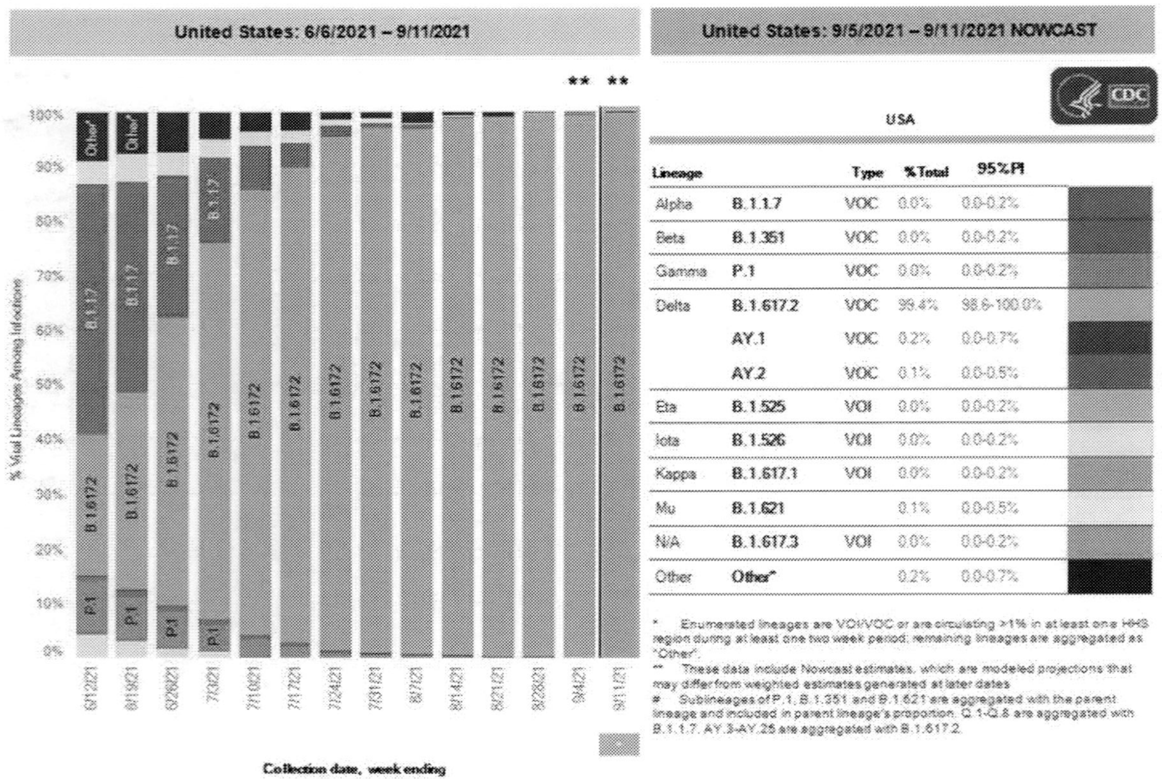

SARS-CoV-2 variants circulating in the United States.

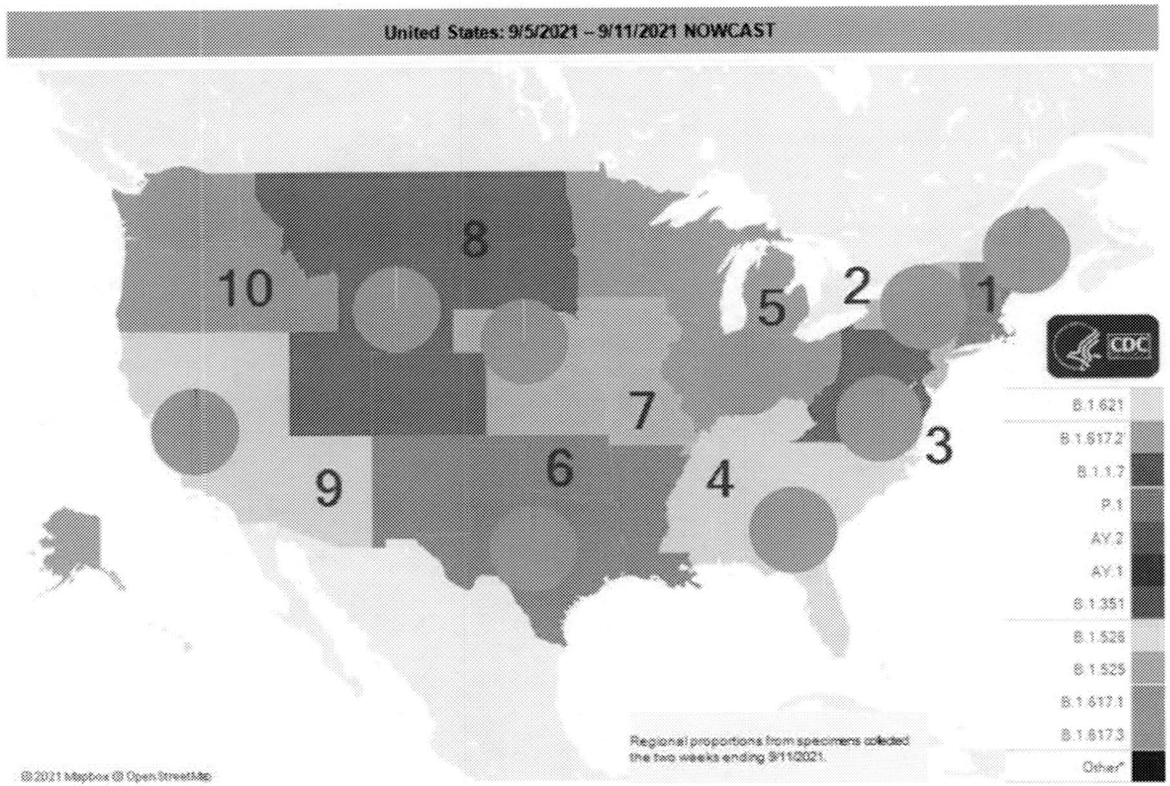

SARS-CoV-2 variants circulating in the United States

Testing

The percentage of COVID-19 NAATs (nucleic acid amplification tests)[4] that are positive (percent positivity) has decreased from the previous week. The 7-day average of percent positivity from NAATs is now 8.9%. The 7-day average number of tests reported for September 3–September 9, 2021, was 1,394,082, down 14.1% from 1,623,346 for the prior 7 days.

Total Tests Reported: 551,805,555
7-Day Average Tests Reported: 1,394,082
7-Day Average % Positivity: 8.9%

Total Tests Reported: 551,805,555
Previous 7-Day Average % Positivity: 9.1%
Change in 7-Day Average % Positivity since Prior Week: -1.8%

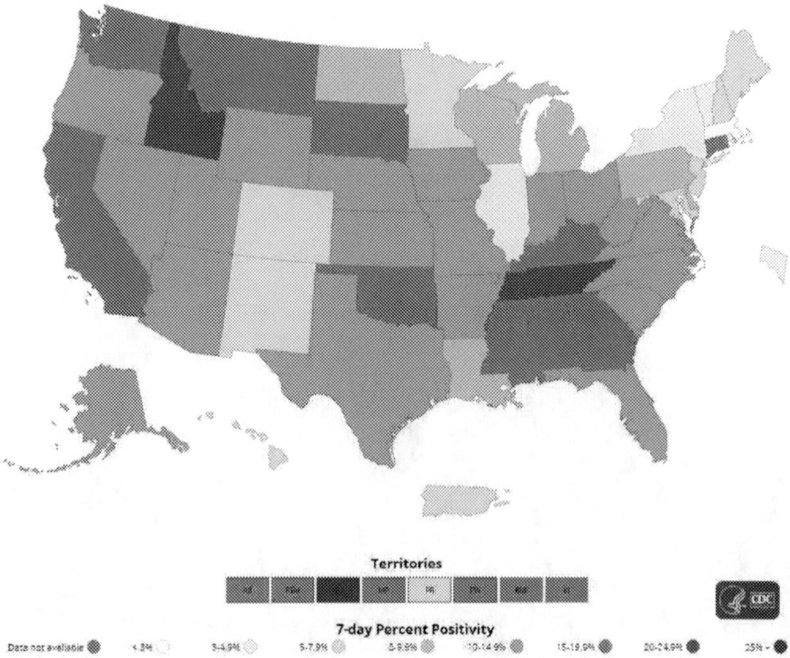

COVID-19 NAAT laboratory test 7-day percent positivity by state/territory.

[4] Test for SARS-CoV-2, the virus that causes COVID-19.

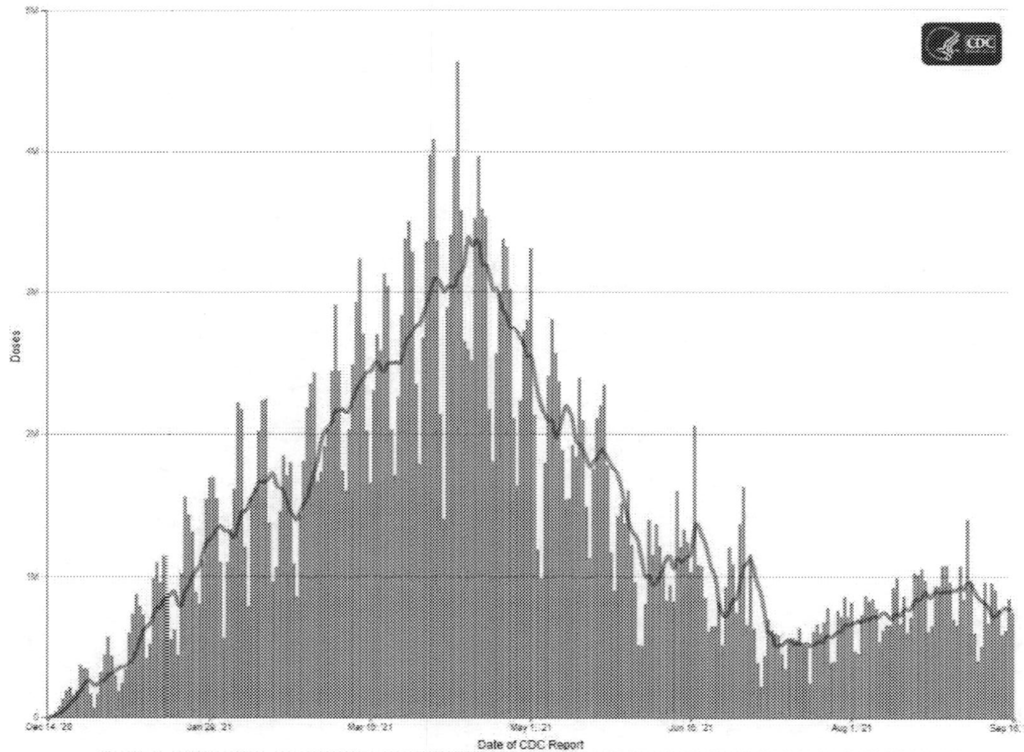

Daily change in the total number of administered COVID-19 vaccine doses reported to CDC by the date of CDC report, United States (red line represents 7-day moving average).

Vaccinations

The U.S. COVID-19 Vaccination Program began December 14, 2020. As of September 16, 2021, 383 million vaccine doses have been administered. Overall, about 210.7 million people, or 63.5% of the total U.S. population, have received at least one dose of vaccine. About 180.1 million people, or 54.2% of the total U.S. population, have been fully vaccinated.[5] As of September 16, 2021, the 7-day average number of administered vaccine doses reported (by date of CDC report) to CDC per day was 773,763, a 1.6% decrease from the previous week.

CDC's COVID Data Tracker Vaccination Demographic Trends tab shows vaccination trends by age group. As of September 16, 2021, 93% of people ages 65 years or older have received at least one dose of vaccine and 82.7% are fully vaccinated. Over three-quarters (76.1%) of people ages 18 years or older have received at least one dose of vaccine and 65.4% are fully vaccinated. For people ages 12 years or older, 74.2% have received at least one dose of vaccine and 63.5% are fully vaccinated.

- Vaccines Administered: 383,038,403
- People who received at least one dose: 210,700,361
- People who are fully vaccinated[6]: 180,086,143
- Percentage of the US population that has received at least one dose: 63.5%
- Percentage of the US population that has been fully vaccinated[7]: 54.2%
- Percentage point increase from last week: +0.8
- Percentage point increase from last week: +0.8

Hospitalizations

New Hospital Admissions

The current 7-day daily average for September 8–September 14, 2021, was 11,165. This is a 5.7% decrease from the prior 7-day average (11,836) from September 1–September 7, 2021.

[5,6,7] Represents the number of people who have received the second dose in a two-dose COVID-19 vaccine series (such as the Pfizer or Moderna vaccines) or one dose of the single-shot Johnson & Johnson's Janssen vaccine.

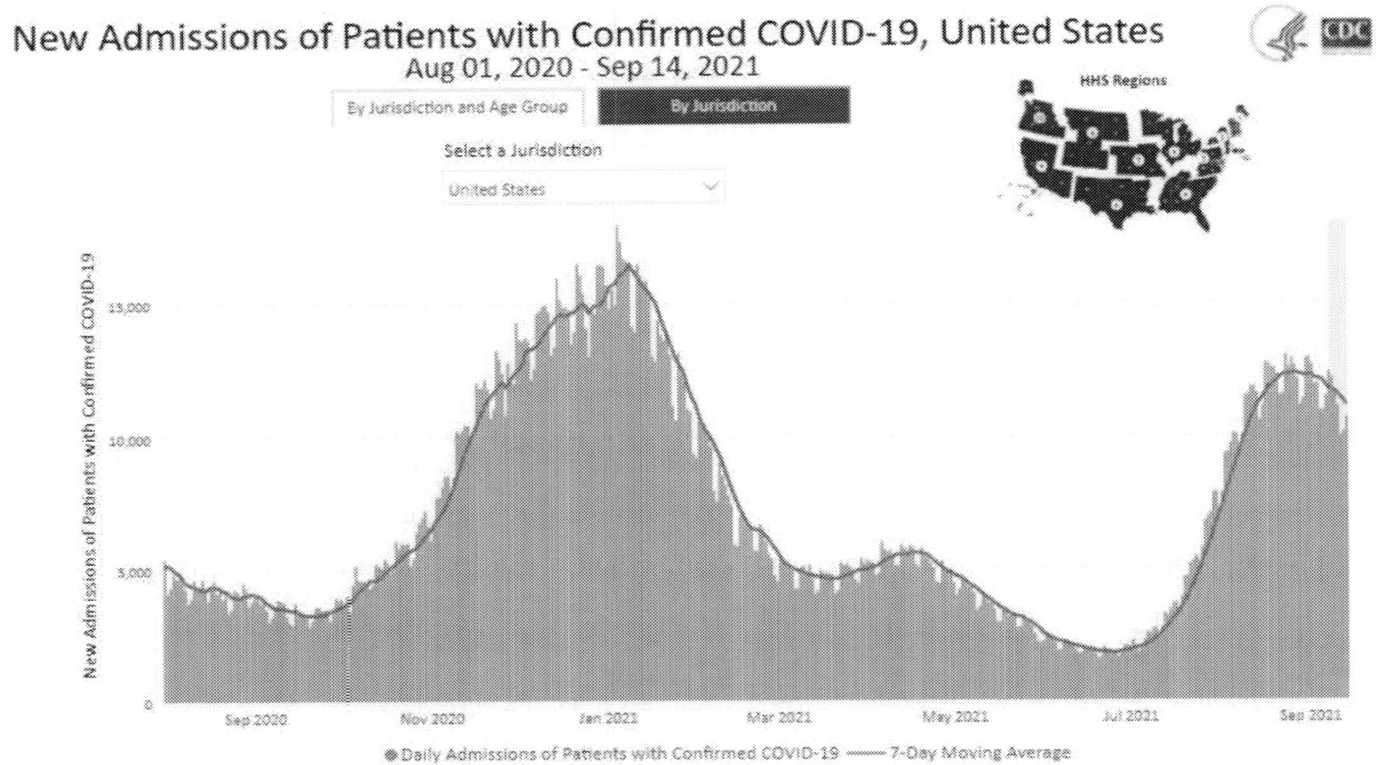

Daily trends in number of New COVID-19 hospital admissions in the United States.

- Total New Admissions: 2,920,532
- Current 7-Day Average: 11,165
- Prior 7-Day Average: 11,836
- Change in 7-Day Average: -5.7%

The start of consistent reporting of hospital admissions data was August 1, 2020.

New admissions are pulled from a 10 am EST snapshot of the HHS Unified Hospital Timeseries Dataset. Due to potential reporting delays, data from the most recent 7 days, as noted in the figure above with the grey bar, should be interpreted with caution. Small shifts in historic data may also occur due to changes in the Centers for Medicare and Medicaid Services (CMS) Provider of Services file, which is used to identify the cohort of included hospitals.

COVID-NET: Trends in Hospitalization Rates in Children Ages 11 Years and Younger Not Eligible for Vaccination

CDC's Coronavirus Disease 2019-Associated Hospitalization Surveillance Network (COVID-NET) shows that hospitalization rates are increasing, including rates in children ages 11 years and younger. Recent weekly rates of COVID-19-associated hospitalizations for these children are the highest they have ever been. Weekly rates in children ages 4 years and younger for the week ending August 28, 2021, are 2.4 per 100,000. Rates in children ages 5–11 years are 0.9 per 100,000 for weeks ending August 9 and August 21, 2021. Unlike adults, children younger than 12 years of age are not yet eligible for any of the available COVID-19 vaccines.

The Coronavirus Disease 2019 (COVID-19)-Associated Hospitalization Surveillance Network (COVID-NET) is an additional source for hospitalization data collected through a network of more than 250 acute-care hospitals in 14 states (representing ~10% of the U.S. population). Detailed data on patient demographics, including race/ethnicity, underlying medical conditions, medical interventions, and clinical outcomes, are standardized case reporting form.

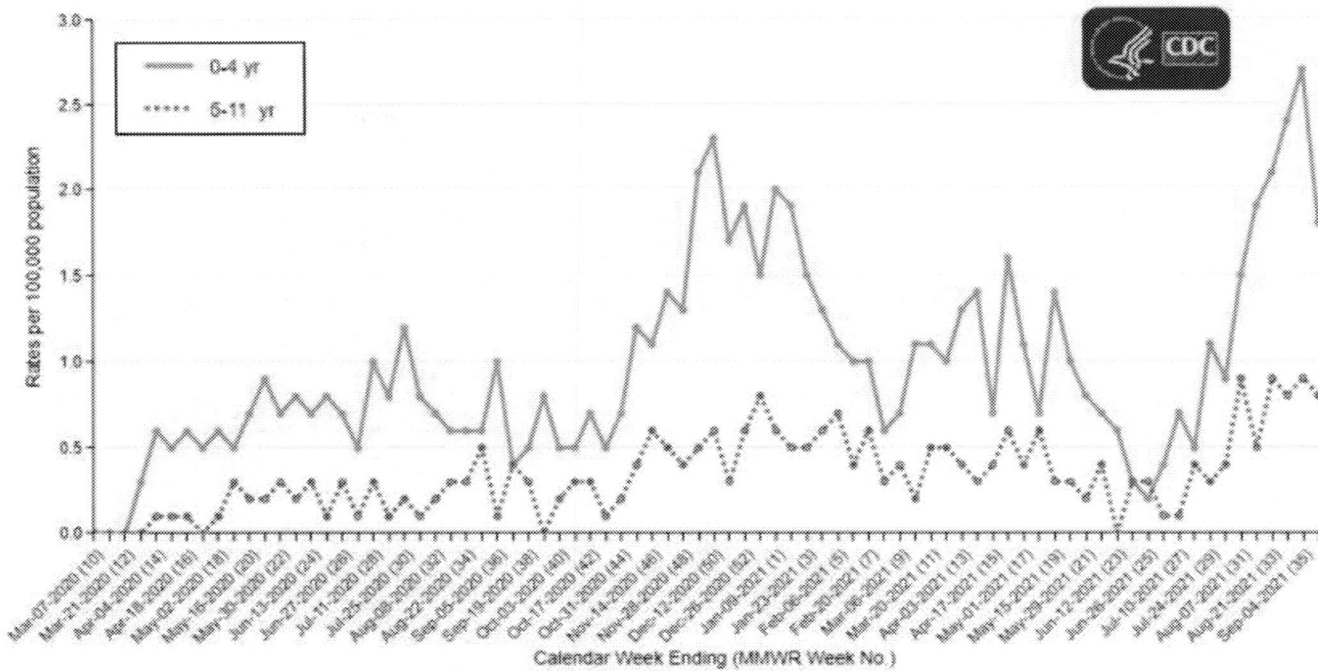

Trends in hospitalization rates in children ages 11 years and younger not eligible for vaccination.

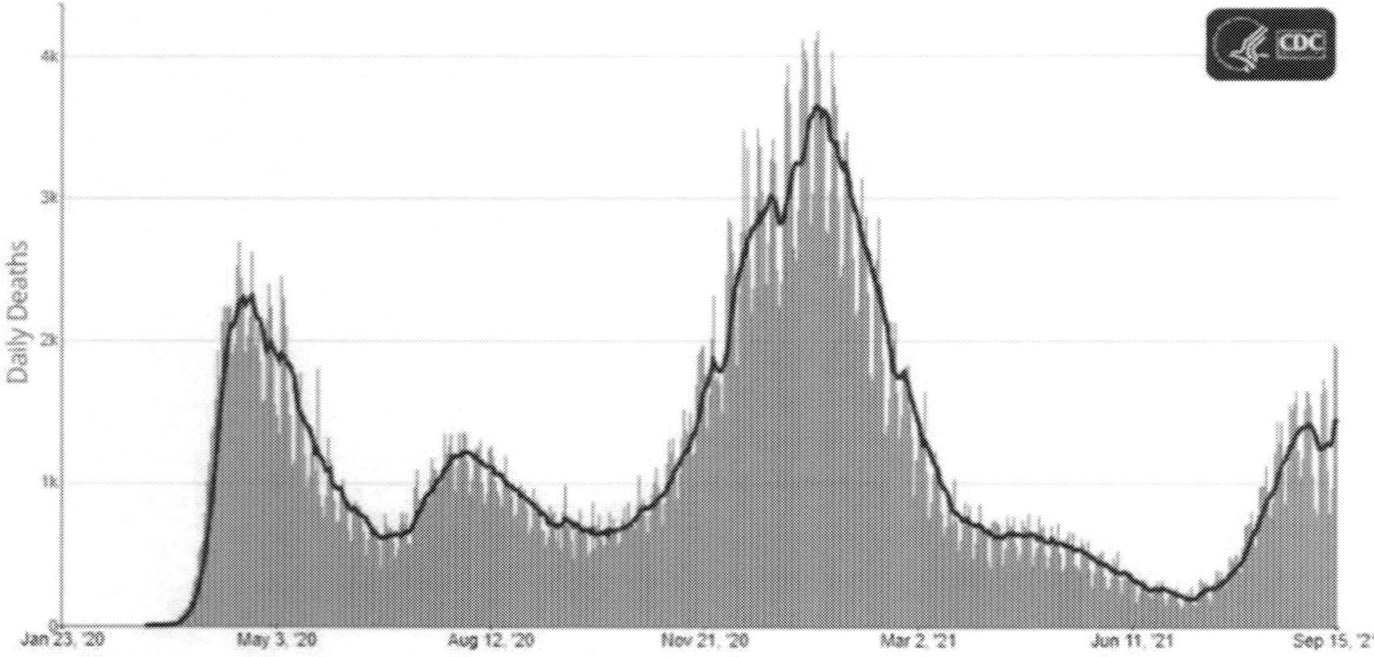

Daily trends in number of COVID-19 deaths in the United States reported to CDC (red line indicated 7-day moving average).

Deaths

The current 7-day moving average of new deaths (1,448) has increased 17.4% compared with the previous 7-day moving average (1,233). As of September 15, 2021, a total of 666,440 COVID-19 deaths have been reported in the United States.

- Total Deaths Reported: 666,440
- Current 7-Day Average[8]: 1,448
- Prior 7-Day Average: 1,233
- Change in 7-Day Average Since Prior Week: 17.4%

[8] Historical deaths are excluded from the daily new deaths and 7-day average calculations until they are incorporated into the dataset by their applicable date. Of 7,633 historical deaths reported retroactively, 202 were reported in the current week and 253 were reported in the prior week.

Chapter 7

A View from the States: Governors Respond to the Omicron Variant*

Committee on Oversight and Reform

Thursday, January 20, 2022
House of Representatives Committee on Oversight and Reform
Select Subcommittee on the Coronavirus Crisis
Washington, D.C.

The subcommittee met, pursuant to notice, at 3:05 p.m., via Zoom, Hon. James E. Clyburn (chairman of the subcommittee) presiding.

Present: Representatives Clyburn, Waters, Maloney, Vela´zquez, Foster, Raskin, Krishnamoorthi, Scalise, Jordan, Malliotakis, and Miller-Meeks.

Chairman CLYBURN. Good afternoon. The committee will come to order.

Without objection, the chair is authorized to declare a recess of the committee at any time.

I now recognize myself for an opening statement.

Since the coronavirus first reached our shores two years ago, governors have played a critical role in responding to the spread of the virus. We are fortunate to be joined today by the Governors of the state of Washington, the state of Colorado, the Commonwealth of Puerto Rico, and the state of Nebraska, as well as the Mayor of the District of Columbia, whose role is equivalent to that of a state governor.

* This is an edited, reformatted and augmented version of Hearing Before the Select Subcommittee on the Coronavirus Crisis of the Committee on Oversight and Reform, House of Representatives, Serial No. 117–62, dated January 20, 2022.

In: A Closer Look at the COVID-19 Variants
Editor: Richard D. Hylton
ISBN: 979-8-88697-170-5

To learn more about the instrumental role, these chief executives continue to play in our Nation's response to the pandemic.

This hearing comes at a pivotal moment in our Nation's response. As we gather today, we are facing new challenges from the highly transmissible Omicron variant, which is resulting in higher case numbers than ever before. However, there is a reason to be hopeful.

Earlier research indicates that Omicron causes less severe disease than previous strands of the coronavirus. We have more effective therapeutics at our disposal than ever to treat the disease. And, most importantly, all approved coronavirus vaccines and boosters continue to provide robust protection against severe disease and death from the Omicron variant.

If you are up-to-date on your coronavirus vaccinations, that is, if you have received your initial shots and then gotten a booster when eligible, you have the protection you need to live your normal life at very low risk to your health and the health of your loved ones.

Unfortunately, the coronavirus pandemic remains a crisis because millions of Americans remain unvaccinated and are therefore at risk of the Omicron variant. Recent data show that unvaccinated Americans continue to account for a substantial majority of hospitalizations and deaths. Given the high transmissibility of the Omicron variant, these unvaccinated patients are pushing many hospital systems to their limits, threatening anyone who may need hospital care.

Many of the Americans who remain unvaccinated have made this dangerous decision because of coronavirus misinformation, which is reaching broad audiences and undermining the great work being done at all levels of government to protect communities from the virus.

Misinformation has also led to fraud too many Americans infected with the coronavirus to reject effective treatments. It is increasingly clear why so many Americans continue to doubt the safety and effectiveness of lifesaving coronavirus vaccines.

Republican politicians are among the most vocal proponents of the misinformation that has generated those doubts. For instance, Senator Ron Johnson stated last year that there had been, and I'm quoting him, over 3,000 deaths within 30 days of taking the vaccine, falsely connecting unrelated deaths to the coronavirus vaccines.

Congressman Matt Gaetz has dangerously encouraged people to get infected, saying, and I'm quoting him, the best vaccine we have found is Mother Nature's vaccine. It's contracting the virus.

Sadly, these are just two of many falsehoods coming from our colleagues across the aisle. Other Republican politicians simply emphasize your right not to be vaccinated, rather than presenting the decision to get vaccinated as the consequential patriotic duty that it is. Because getting vaccinated doesn't just protect yourself; it protects your loved ones, your communities, and your fellow citizens.

The ranking member of this committee has criticized the Biden administration's vaccine requirements as, and I'm quoting, increasing government control of your life, end of quote. This type of discouragement is legitimizing and perpetrating people's vaccine hesitance when we should be working together to vaccinate as many Americans as possible.

The Republican Party's promotion of misinformation has measurable consequences. One study found that political affiliation is the strongest predictor of whether someone is vaccinated, with unvaccinated adults more than three times as likely to lean Republican as Democrat. Since vaccines became widely available in May 2021, people living in counties that voted heavily for former President Trump in 2020 were three times as likely to die from the coronavirus as those who lived in areas that voted for President Biden. The irresponsible legitimization of vaccine misinformation by Republican leaders is tragically killing their supporters.

This vaccine resistance is among the top challenges facing leaders at the Federal and state levels as we enter 2022 at the height of the Omicron wave. I look forward to hearing from today's witnesses to further understand how the Federal Government can work with states, territories, and the District of Columbia to overcome vaccine hesitancy, combat the Omicron variant, and prepare for any further challenges this virus may present.

The past two years have shown that Federal-state collaboration is critical to mounting an effective response to the coronavirus. We saw the dire consequences of the Trump administration's abdication of Federal leadership and refusal to provide support to states in acquiring and distributing critical personal protective equipment, tests, and other supplies during the first year of the pandemic, forcing states to fend for themselves.

Since taking office, President Biden has emphasized the importance of working with the states, territories, and the District of Columbia to respond to the pandemic.

Under Governor Inslee's leadership, Washington State recently set up a mobile vaccination unit in King County with capacity to administer up to 1,500 vaccines and booster shots per day, and is working to set up another high-capacity site.

Under Governor Polis, Colorado recently worked with FEMA to set up mobile bus units to administer monoclonal antibody treatments in rural areas of the state, congregate living facilities, and other high-demand sites.

Under Governor Pierluisi, Puerto Rico has worked hard to build vaccine confidence and get shots in arms, with result that nearly 80 percent of Puerto Ricans are fully vaccinated—one of the highest vaccination rates among the United States and its territories. Using funds from the American Rescue Act, Mayor Bowser and the District of Columbia have helped families struggling with rent and housing security during the pandemic. Of course, Washington, DC.'s lack of statehood status has impacted the District's response. Republicans refuse to provide the District with $755 million in relief funding via the CARES Act that it would have been entitled to if it were a state.

Now, I'm particularly concerned about this because this is not just people; these are Americans living in our Nation's Capital. They are family members. Scores of my family members left South Carolina and went to Washington, DC, Philadelphia, New York, other places looking to further—get further access to the greatness of America. And to be penalized living in the District of Columbia is just beyond the pale. These people are American citizens and should have been treated better. Fortunately, Congress restored this funding, and the Biden administration, in the American Rescue Act.

I would like to thank today's witnesses for taking the time to testify about these pressing issues. I look forward to hearing from our Governors about their responses to the Omicron variant and gaining more insight into how we can better protect Americans and end this crisis.

I now recognize the ranking member for his opening statement.

Mr. SCALISE. Thank you, Mr. Chairman. I look forward to hearing from our witnesses.

I want to start by making it very clear for those of us who have promoted the vaccine, who have talked about what President Trump started under Operation Warp Speed to create, not one, buttwo, but three vaccines. The real flaw—and there have been many flaws with President Biden's approach—has been to have a vaccine-only strategy where he's tried to shame people based on whether or not they get the vaccine, trying to divide people on whether or not they get the vaccine.

It's misinformation to suggest only unvaccinated are dying or only Republicans or Trump voters are dying. There is clearly all throughout our country right now a resurgence in COVID. Affects blue states, red states, Republicans, Democrats, Black, White, Hispanic, Asian.

What we should be focused on is how to confront it. Unfortunately, if you look where we are today, today marks the one-year anniversary that Joe Biden took the oath of office as President of the United States. Unfortunately, what we've seen is failure after failure and broken promise after broken promise. And, unfortunately, it starts with the vaccine and what President Biden said he would do about COVID and has failed to do a year in.

He promised Americans that he would, quote, shut down the virus. How many times did we hear Joe Biden say that, promise that as a candidate? Unfortunately, what we're going to see is a very different candidate Joe Biden versus President Joe Biden. Words versus actions.

Shut down the virus was what he promised. Yet despite inheriting all three of those proven, safe, and effective vaccines from President Trump's Operation Warp Speed, as well as numerous proven treatments, therapeutics. Millions of people, by the way, with natural immunity, which, Mr. Chairman, we ought to have a hearing about to see just what kind of protection natural immunity gives people.

He also had a well-established testing apparatus that he walked into. Right now, the United States, with all of that, is being hit with record highs for new cases. Testing shortages and delays. And there have been more deaths under Joe Biden's Presidency than under Donald Trump's. Again, a year in, and he walked in the door with three vaccines ready to go. President Trump didn't have any of that.

And I know there's been a lot of talk under the Trump administration about how many deaths there were by Democrats. Interesting you don't hear them talking about the deaths right now, that Joe Biden has more deaths under his Presidency than we had under Trump.

A signature feature of then-candidate Biden's campaign was a top-down Federal solution to the pandemic. How many times did we hear him say that he had a national plan, he was ready to go. On August 18 of 2020, he said, quote, Donald Trump still doesn't have a plan to get this virus under control. His failure to lead is costing American lives.

On October 15 of 2020, he said, quote, What, eight months into this pandemic and Donald Trump still doesn't have a plan to get this virus under control. I do.

That was Joe Biden as a candidate.

Never mind the fact that President Trump had a very successful plan. It was called Operation Warp Speed. It was a bipartisan effort, by the way, in Congress that helped fund Operation WarpSpeed. It should have been bipartisan credit where everybody bragged about the success of Operation

Warp Speed. It yielded those three safe and effective vaccines. It yielded multiple therapies like monoclonal antibodies. And we had a robust testing network.

On President Biden's first day in office, he released a 200-page document titled, quote, National Strategy for the COVID–19 Response and Pandemic Preparedness. And he said, quote, For the past year, we could not turn to the Federal Government for a national plan to answer prayers with action until today.

Well, just a few weeks ago, in a stunning reversal, after almost a year of broken promises and failed strategy, and the virus raging worse than ever before, President Biden reversed course and abandoned that so-called plan.

On December 27 of 2021, just a few weeks ago, President Biden said, quote, there is no Federal solution. This gets solved at the state level. I am guessing that's why the select subcommittee is having this hearing today, titled, "A View from the States."

After campaigning on a national plan and congressional Democrats, including many on this committee, calling for a national plan, Democrats have now abandoned any hint of a plan and instead are trying to dump their failures into the Governors' laps.

Ironically, President Biden's first goal in his national strategy was to, quote, restore trust with the American people. Yet his policy shows he does not trust the American people. He does not trust the American people enough to be transparent about the policies and decisions his administration is making and the data that they are using to make those decisions. He does not trust the American people to make their own healthcare decisions. He does not trust the healthcare workers to make their own healthcare decisions.

Interestingly, if you look a year ago, we were all praising healthcare workers, unvaccinated healthcare workers as heroes. Today, President Biden is trying to fire those very same healthcare workers if they're unvaccinated.

What changed in a year? Why were they heroes a year ago and today President Biden wants those same people to be fired? Talk about trusting the American people.

He doesn't trust parents to make decisions about what's best for their children. He does not trust businesses to make decisions about what's best for the welfare of their employees. Trust is a two- way street, and this is but one reason why President Biden's COVID response plan is in tatters. Instead of trying to patch the holes in the Biden administration's messaging, this subcommittee should be fulfilling its stated purpose; that is, performing congressional oversight of the COVID–19 response.

The list of issues that we should be having hearings on is incredibly long. And, Mr. Chairman, you know, because I've asked many times, that this committee do get engaged in having hearings on some of the oversight that we're not doing. I'll just name a few that we've been calling on this committee to deal with.

The Biden administration's inaction with procuring tests, and rejection of a plan that was reported last October was provided to President Biden to provide millions—hundreds of millions of rapid tests in time for the Christmas holidays. President Biden, by all reports, rejected that plan.

Americans are still wondering, did the President have that plan presented to him? Did he reject it? Who was involved in rejecting that plan and why? And, also, importantly, who's been held accountable if that really did happen? This committee should be getting to the bottom of that.

President Biden's plan of shaming and blaming the unvaccinated instead of focusing on a science-driven approach, to include not only vaccinations but natural immunity, other therapeutics. Stop dividing Americans over the vaccine and start providing Americans with an actual plan to confront this.

The Biden administration commandeered the distribution of monoclonal antibodies, causing states to jump through more hoops and making it harder for states to get access to these lifesaving treatments. We hear from states who are now being forced to compete against other states, and some states aren't being given what they need while others are. That's going on right now under President Biden.

Despite spending about $200 billion to safely reopen schools, more than 5,000 schools have had some type of shutdown this month. Why isn't every school open? We've heard from scientists who said they all should be. Kids are much better off in the classroom.

We need to have a hearing to examine the severe student learning loss caused by remote and hybrid learning. We've heard about the mental health crises that's been caused by students not being allowed to be in a classroom. And, by the way, if a school took the money, like Chicago taking $2 billion of taxpayer money to reopen and then closed their doors on those same students, shouldn't those schools have to give the taxpayer money back? Let's talk about having a hearing to give parents options to send their kids to an open school if their school doesn't want to educate their kids but wants to take the money.

And let's not forget that the teachers' union was caught manipulating CDC guidance on school reopenings. We should have a hearing on manipulating the science that happened by teachers' unions in the Biden White House.

The World Health Organization and the European Center for Disease Prevention and Control do not recommend masking kids under six years old. Why is America masking kids without evidence, and what impact is it having on their emotional and social development? What could be more important than protecting our kids' mental health which has been under attack this last year and a half?

The Biden administration has been sidelining the science on boosters. First, in the summer of 2021, the Biden administration announced the availability of booster shots for all adults by September. But amazingly, they made this announcement before the FDA and the CDC had even finished reviewing the data to determine the need for booster shots. Because of this, two senior FDA officials reportedly left the agency amid alarming reports of political interference with the science under the Biden administration.

This was obviously very confusing for the public. Misinformation clearly by the Biden administration.

Most recently, President Biden's administration chose to add to the confusion by bypassing the FDA and CDC's long-established vaccine advisory committee process for updating booster shot eligibility.

Then, there's the Biden's Operation Snail Speed on Covid Therapies, as The Wall Street Journal editorial board called it. Instead of taking a multifaceted approach to ending the pandemic, President Biden went all in on vaccine-only approach and neglected to focus on therapeutics and natural immunity.

In fact, one year after taking office, President Biden still to this day does not have an FDA Commissioner in place. That should have been a day-one decision. President Biden a year and still doesn't have anybody heading up the FDA. And many people have called the FDA a rudderless ship on things like testing, alternative therapeutics.

Republicans on the select subcommittee still are the only ones in Congress that have held a hearing on the origins of COVID–19. We've asked, Mr. Chairman, that this committee, the full committee have a hearing on the origins.

We've seen a lot of scientific data out there that it started in the lab in Wuhan. There are even reports that some of Dr. Fauci's own advisors said that it started in the lab in Wuhan, and then amazingly days later reversed course. Shouldn't we have a hearing on that? Did somebody interfere with the science to make those scientists reverse course from emails that were hidden and just became public?

The U.S. appears to have funded gain-of-function research at the Wuhan lab in China. Taxpayers should know the truth about that. And we should have a debate and discussion about whether we should be funding those types of research if that was the case.

And, last, newly released unredacted emails, as I talked about regarding Dr. Fauci and Dr. Collins, say that they were warned that COVID–19 came from the lab. We need to do our jobs and look into all of these items. This country spent, through Congress, over $6 trillion of taxpayer money, some of it directly on COVID relief. Some of it was directed into other places that had nothing to do with COVID. But we should be having oversight into all of that.

If we sit idly by as the Biden administration keeps fumbling this pandemic response, then things will only get worse.

Americans want accountability, Mr. Chairman. Let's have hearings to get to the bottom of all of these crises that have been created by this President's failed response to the pandemic.

Look forward to hearing from our witnesses, and I yield back.

Chairman CLYBURN. I thank the ranking member for his remarks.

I would like now to introduce our distinguished witnesses.

Governor Jared Polis, a former colleague, has served as Governor of Colorado since 2019. Governor Polis has taken bold action to lead his state through the pandemic, working tirelessly to ensure children and teachers can attend school in person safely. His administration has distributed millions of medical-grade masks and also onsite vaccine clinics at schools. I would expect no less from a former colleague.

Governor Pierluisi, also a former colleague, has served as Governor of Puerto Rico since 2021. Under his leadership, the Commonwealth of Puerto Rico has worked tirelessly to educate residents about the importance of vaccinations, helping to achieve one of the highest vaccinated mission rates and one of the lowest death rates in the country. His administration has also implemented effective testing and contact tracing efforts, helping to slow the spread of the virus while sustaining Puerto Rico's vital tourism industry.

Mayor Muriel Bowser has served as the Mayor of the District of Columbia since 2015. She has recently overseen an expansive effort to provide residents free at-home testing kits and established multiple coronavirus centers around the city dedicated to expanding access to vaccines and testing. Mayor Bowser's administration has also implemented commonsense vaccine requirements which will save countless lives.

Governor Pete Ricketts has served as Governor of Nebraska since 2015. He has developed a fantastic reputation as one who is compassionate and sensitive to what needs to be done to get beyond this pandemic. He also currently serves as a co-chair of the Republican Governors Association.

Another of my former colleagues and congressional classmate, Governor Jay Inslee, has served as Governor of Washington since 2013. Governor Inslee showed tremendous leadership in responding to one of the earliest coronavirus outbreaks in the country in February 2020, helping to slow the spread of the virus and save lives. Governor Inslee's administration continues to take action to expand access to testing, increase vaccinations, and distribute masks to the public for free.

Now I would like for the witnesses, please, raise your right hands.

Do you swear or affirm that the testimony you're about to give is the truth, the whole truth, and nothing but the truth, so help you God?

Let the record show that the witnesses answered in the affirmative.

Without objection, their written statements will be made part of the record.

Governor Polis, you are now recognized for five minutes for your opening statement.

Statement of Governor Jared Polis, State of Colorado

Mr. POLIS. Thank you, Chairman Clyburn, Ranking Member Scalise. It is good to see my friends and former colleagues and an honor to be invited to share Colorado's experience fighting the COVID–19 pandemic.

Over the last two years, we have relied on data and science to guide our response to the virus. We have taken a balanced approach, prioritizing the health and safety of our fellow Coloradans, working to lessen the psychological and social impact of the pandemic, while minimizing any negative impact on the economy or on our kids' education.

This has led Colorado to have one of the shortest shutdown stay- at-home periods in the entire country. One of the lowest death rates in the entire country as well in the bottom 10 states.

When the lifesaving vaccine became available, we aggressively launched efforts to protect as many Coloradans who wanted to be protected. We were proud that we vaccinated 70 percent of Coloradans by—70 and older—early on. And we reached President Biden's goal of vaccinating 70 percent of all Coloradans by July 4. And we brought that same intensity to protecting our kids, our 5- to 11-year-olds, as well as administering third doses shown to be even more important against the Omicron variant.

The lifesaving vaccine is our single best tool against the virus, especially against severe illness and death from the virus. But early detection also helps prevent the disease spread, and through more and more effective treatments, also save lives. And that's why we have worked to make testing free, quick, and easy. Over 100 community testing sites.

Last year, we made rapid tests available through an at-home delivery program that continues to this day. We're really thrilled to see a similar national home test delivery program rolled out as well. And we're happy to see the Federal Government step up in that regard.

We also used testing to protect state employees, working with many of the vulnerable workers under our care, including at veterans' nursing homes, youth detention facilities. And we worked with schools to make free testing available onsite for students and staff to help improve the level of safety in the classroom.

Earlier this week, Colorado launched a new mask delivery program that provides free medical-grade masks to every Coloradan who wants them. They are at dozens of public libraries, fire stations, recreation centers, YMCA's, depots that have agreed to be part of a distribution hub. And Coloradans can pick up five medical-grade masks to add additional protection to themselves.

These programs are examples of how we've worked to tackle the virus from every angle. I'm very proud of everyday Americans, everyday Coloradans, the way that they have stepped up to protect themselves and their family during this crisis. But the simple truth is that states alone cannot spearhead these efforts indefinitely. COVID–19 is no doubt with us for years to come. And while early data suggests we're entering the endemic phases of this virus soon, we should also be prepared for the inevitable lulls and subsequent waves that will continue to impact hospital capacity as well as, of course, the threat of future mutations.

Protecting hospital capacity has always been our North Star in Colorado. We wanted to make sure that if anybody gets a heart attack, a stroke, a car accident, or sick with COVID has access to the very best care to make sure that they can recover. What we simply cannot allow how we live and work and how our children go to school to be determined by whether or not our hospitals can keep up or hire staff or maintain adequate supplies.

We need a national standard of hospital and healthcare system readiness. And we know that with the disruptions in the work force, especially in healthcare, like people across the country, we're losing many nurses, doctors, and staff, and we need national focus on a plan to improve work force readiness around the healthcare work force for the future.

Colorado is working on a plan with our providers, with legislators to invest in our healthcare work force, but we can't stand alone. This truly needs to be a national effort.

It's not just about the need for hospital beds and workers; it's also about integrating the pandemic response as an endemic response into our healthcare system where it belongs.

Colorado, of course, like many states, set up testing sites, vaccine clinics, distributed therapeutics. But moving forward, our medical system—doctors, pharmacies, urgent cares, hospitals—should be providing this care, as they do for all other conditions.

Coloradans trust their primary care doctors and turn to them first. But because FEMA is not reimbursing costs associated with equipping primary care and pediatric physicians to provide vaccines, many doctors are still not offering this critical protection to their patients, putting a further onus on the states and, of course, hospitals and pharmacies.

Similarly, far too many schools in Colorado and across the country don't have a designated school nurse; someone to administer tests onsite, take temperatures, catch cases in their infancy. But because of this, we see a lot of outbreaks and children needlessly getting sick and contributing to their family members getting sick who might be more vulnerable.

Colorado has worked to get schools the supplies they need, including masking. We've distributed over 2 million masks to teachers, as well as to students, at school and onsite testing. But both, of course, are opt-in programs. And we need our schools to have on- site, high-quality care to make sure the kids get the uninterrupted safe education they deserve.

We know what we need do. It's going to take all of us working together to get it done.

I want to thank Chairman Clyburn. I want to thank the subcommittee for inviting me here today. I hope that this perspective from Colorado can help spur national action to help our country move forward, protect lives, and keep our economy growing.

And I yield back.

Chairman CLYBURN. Thank you very much, Governor Polis.

We'll now hear from Governor Pierluisi. Governor, you are now recognized for five minutes.

Statement of Governor Pedro Pierluisi, Commonwealth of Puerto Rico

Mr. PIERLUISI. Chairman Clyburn, Ranking Member Scalise, and members of the subcommittee, thank you for inviting me to testify before you today.

As Governor of Puerto Rico and former resident commissioner of Puerto Rican Congress, I'm honored to represent the unique viewpoint of the island's 3.2 million American citizens as we enter the third year of this pandemic.

When my administration took office in January 2021, I put together a team of highly qualified professionals and scientists to advise me on how to lead our fight against COVID–19. We worked tirelessly to educate our citizens on the value of the vaccine, which bolstered vaccine uptake and staved off skepticism. Because of these efforts, over 91.4 percent of our vaccine-eligible population over the age of 5 have received at least one dose, and an astounding 81.5 percent of our vaccine-eligible population is fully vaccinated or boosted. Puerto Rico stands as the leader in the Nation's vaccination effort.

An important aspect of Puerto Rico's successful vaccine rollout was the connectivity amongst the healthcare providers on the island. When monoclonal antibody treatments became widely available, thanks to the hard work of HHS, Puerto Rico leaned heavily on our strong pharmacy networks to ensure that there was a coordinated request for therapeutics needed each week.

Puerto Rico engineered one of the first electronic vaccine card programs in the United States, the VacuID. Our department of health, led by Dr. Carlos Mellado, deployed strong contact tracing teams and effectively monitored visitors, identified positive COVID patients, and slowed the spread. These efforts enabled us to sustain much of our tourism industry, an important component of Puerto Rico's economy.

Puerto Rico is regularly asked to do more with less. However, with the right leadership and depoliticization of healthcare, our island stands as proof that it is possible to achieve successful outcomes. We can only envision just how resilient our island could be if there was less disparity in Federal funding for our healthcare programs.

When treated equally with the states, as we have been for much of the COVID-related Federal disbursements, Puerto Rico has been able to accomplish a high standard of care for the citizens of our territory. We have been able to achieve the near impossible, having no hospitals closing their doors during the COVID–19 pandemic.

Over the last two years, while cases have spiked in the U.S. and around the world, we have been able to keep Puerto Rico's case counts comparatively low. However, with the rise of the Delta and Omicron variants, we have seen the highest case counts reported to date. We have had approximately 239,000 confirmed cases recorded on the island, with our daily case count continuing to decline now to less than 2,000 confirmed cases per day. Throughout the pandemic, we have had 3,593 confirmed deaths due to COVID– 19, with our daily average continuing to decrease. These numbers are comparatively low due to our high rates of vaccination.

However, given that we are an island, the possibility of overburdening our health system has always been a concern, as our people cannot be diverted to a neighboring state hospital. My administration has been very proactive and creative with mandates through- out this pandemic. Since midsummer of 2021, we have required most of our work force to be fully vaccinated. Although we have always given our citizens the option to provide negative COVID test results in lieu of proof of vaccination, we have continuously advocated for vaccination across all sectors of our society.

In addition, we have not been shy about requiring restaurants and bars to ask for proof of vaccination or a negative test result to their clients at all times. And every time we have faced spikes in cases, we have promptly restricted both capacity and business hours at our gastronomic and entertainment venues.

As the U.S.' most populous territory, Puerto Rico's differential treatment in total healthcare programs creates gaps in the services we can provide our citizens.

While Congress passed legislation to increase Puerto Rico's Federal medical assistance percent, the FMAP in the Medicaid program from 55 percent up to 76 percent, that number has been allowed to lapse since the December 3 CR. This unanticipated reversion to a lower FMAP percentage has triggered severe consequences on the island, potentially causing newly enrolled Medicaid beneficiaries to lose their health coverage if this is not addressed.

As the February 18 government funding deadline approaches, I urge this subcommittee to work with your colleagues to set Puerto Rico's FMAP to at least 76 percent.

Sustained progress is made difficult by short-term or altogether insufficient funding. I mention this because it emphasizes the mountain we in Puerto Rico must climb when responding to any health crisis. We must lift ourselves to equal footing with states that have just as many American citizens to care for.

I assure you that with the Federal funding, Puerto Rico can prosper and continue to provide Americans a safe place to invest in, visit, and live.

Thank you, and I look forward to answering any questions you may have.

Chairman CLYBURN. Thank you, Governor. The chair now recognizes Mayor Bowser.

Statement of Mayor Muriel Bowser, District of Columbia

Ms. BOWSER. Thank you, Mr. Chairman. And I want to thank the ranking member as well. And I am delighted to present Washington, D.C.'s experience with our COVID response. We have prepared a few slides to go through our response and recovery from COVID.

Are you able to see those?

And like my colleagues who have already presented, I am grateful to the outstanding team that has supported our response in the District, led by Dr. LaQuandra Nesbitt at D.C. Health, and Chris Rodriguez at D.C. HSEMA. They have led 37,000 D.C. government employees and grateful residents, businesses, and visitors in the District.

We are showing here our experience over the four waves of COVID and how we focused on six pillars of D.C.'s COVID response—we can advance the slide—to flatten the curve—we can go to the next slide—being the first charge to D.C. residents.

How we have focused on proven public health interventions throughout these four phases, including what the tools that have been at our disposal as chief executives, including from in early days relying on stay-at-home orders, masking, social distancing requirements and, of course, very timely community health guidance, travel advisories, and now vaccine requirements throughout several sectors in the city.

We have also been very focused on our testing and vaccination capability. I'm very proud. I call it the gold standard of testing that we've been able to set up throughout our pandemic response. Including on tapping into other first responders, we set up PCR testing at our firehouses early in the pandemic. We've also called on our libraries to be distribution points for our at-home testing and now our rapid test distribution.

We have conducted in our city over 800,000 tests that are walk- up testing sites. And since this surge in Omicron, we have distributed 329,000 free rapid tests to D.C. residents since December 2021.

We also are proud that D.C. residents are getting vaccinated, but we know we continue to have work to do, and so we are still coming up with new strategies to get more people vaxxed and boosted. We also know that the work that we have done in our human services helped us bend the curve and save lives among our most vulnerable residents, including those who are experiencing home- lessness, by setting up isolation and quarantine hotels and alternate accommodations for people who have high-risk health conditions.

And that work, I must say, has been aided by a very abled FEMA who worked hand-in-hand with us to make sure that those pretty significant expenditures would qualify for reimbursement.

Contact tracing has been a key part of the work that we have done. And we hired over 500 people to get that work done.

And we have also—next slide—been very focused as it has been key to our work with COVID at giving our residents direct, timely, accurate information and dispelling any misinformation that's out there. We have done that, front and center, with situational updates that I have delivered on a pretty frequent cadence. We have experienced significant views on our website of people wanting to follow the data and listen to the science so that they can make decisions that keep their families safe.

We're also very proud of the work that we did door-to-door. You will hear a number of us talk about how to deal with misinformation and give people—get people to make the decision to get vaccinated. And we did that by empowering a community Ambassador corps. So, neighbor-to-neighbor conversations to get people vaccinated. And we knocked over a quarter of a million doors to do exactly that.

Next slide.

We, of course, have been focused on making sure our healthcare system could support, of course, flattening the curve until the vaccines were available and distributed, and they were able do that. And now, we are also working to make sure that the system can support this Omicron variant that we've experienced the last several weeks and anything else that we will see with COVID as the months go on.

We, as has been mentioned, established community COVID centers which are in retail spaces that will give D.C. Health some permanent space to work out of as we try to advance our vaccine and booster strategy. Residents will also be able to go to those locations for testing kits, masks, and to ask questions.

We have, throughout the pandemic, as I mentioned, also supported a huge testing program where we use firehouses and our libraries. And we've partnered with our faith communities, especially in hesitant communities throughout the District.

Gratefully, we did not have to use our 430 seven-bed alternate care site, but we did set that up in the case that we had an influx in the early days of the pandemic.

Next, we have been very focused on all of our social services as well, and that should be emphasized throughout this. No chief executive wants to shut down her city, send people home from work and school and away from their doctors and other trusted individuals that can help with nutrition, emergency commodities, and family assistance in a lot of areas.

We did—D.C. residents did—we lost over 1,200 of our residents to COVID. And many of them were able to take advantage of the funeral assistance offered by FEMA.

We also were very quick in getting our dollars out that came through the American Rescue Plan for rental assistance. Keeping people in housing during this emergency has been one of our top priorities. We distributed $352 million in our STAY D.C. program, and more than 50,000 families received assistance.

So, as we talk about what the Federal Government will continue to be called on to do, we know that the economic crisis that COVID created is going to have some long tails, and so we want to make sure that we're paying attention to that.

And, next, I just mentioned the types of things that it takes for a government to pivot on a dime to transition to remote work, to make sure that our facilities are safe for children to return to school and workers to return. We were very proud that our government, 37,000 D.C. government employees returned to in-person work in July 2021.

You're going to, Mr. Chairman, hear us talk about another thing that the Federal Government can do, and that's get back to in-person work in the Nation's Capitol as well. And so we'll continue to talk about ways that Federal agencies can implement their return- to-work strategies.

We also were able, as I mentioned, to work hand-in-hand with you, Mr. Chairman, and other Members of the Congress to restore $755 million in CARES Act funding that the District was shorted. And that is very important to how we were able to implement all the testing strategies and responses to COVID that we've been able to do.

Next slide.

And we also have some—we put this in the category of unexpected things that have happened as we were also responding to COVID. Our city was still running. All of the things that happened in cities were happening. We, of course, in the District had to deal with large-scale First Amendment protests in the summer of 2020 that consumed a lot of our emergency resources and police resources. We, of course, responded to support the United States Capitol Police on January 6 and supported the inauguration of 2021.

We continue to be in a posture where we can respond to these variants and any variants that come in the future. We should also not forget that we had a very active hurricane season in 2020. So, I mention those things because the strain on our response, emergency response, first responders and police in the summer of 2020 was very significant.

We are——

Chairman CLYBURN. Mayor Bowser? Ms. BOWSER. Yes.

Chairman CLYBURN. You've gone far beyond the five minutes.

Ms. BOWSER. OK. Let me just say, finally, Mr. Chairman, that the return to school has been a priority for us. We like others have dealt with Omicron. We saw, we think, our daily cases peak at the end of December or first part of January. And now we see all of our daily metrics improving from weekly case rate, daily case rate, hospitalizations, and all of the—and even our vaccination numbers improving as we speak.

Chairman CLYBURN. Well, thank you very much, Mayor Bowser. Ms. BOWSER. Thank you.

Chairman CLYBURN. I feel that all those who have some questions, you may expand at that time.

It is now my pleasure to recognize Governor Ricketts. Governor Ricketts, you're recognized for five minutes.

Statement of Governor Pete Ricketts, State of Nebraska

Mr. RICKETTS. Thank you very much, Chairman Clyburn, Ranking Member Scalise, members of the committee. I appreciate the opportunity to be here today. It's an honor.

My name is Pete Ricketts, and I am the Governor of the state of Nebraska. And as has been pointed out already, the COVID virus and pandemic has changed the way we do business, where we learn, the way we go about our daily life. And through it all, Nebraskans have done the right thing, they've taken care of themselves and come through this strong.

In fact, one of the recent demonstrations of this was a Politico report that looked at the state pandemic response. And across four areas, including health, social well-being, education, and economy, Nebraska came out ranked No. 1 as far as overall best response to the pandemic.

And this really goes back to how it all started for us. We got some great advice early on from the officials at University of Nebraska Medical Center who told me, Hey, there's a virus. You can't stop it. You can only slow it down until you can buildup the resources to fight it, and you have to protect your hospital capacity. So, along that line, we were one of the first states to focused on hospital capacity as driving all of our pandemic response. And it's been true from the moment this started back in March 2020 to today.

So, we put together a seven-point plan to be able to address the pandemic. The first started with create testing capacity. We set up TestNebraska, which more than doubled our testing capacity here in the state. We hired over a thousand contact tracers to supplement our local public health departments and their efforts. We purchased PPE for our hospitals and first responders and anybody else who needed it. In fact, we were one of the first states or the first state to have 120 days' worth of PPE on supply.

We also created a quarantine space for folks who couldn't go home for whatever reason, using dormitory rooms or hotels so that we wouldn't have people spreading the virus.

We focused on at-risk communities, long-term care facilities, or meat processing, with additional attention to make sure in those congregate settings we were reducing the risk of spreading it.

And then, of course, we had our directed health measures which put restrictions in place early on, such as limiting restaurants to have only carryouts and so forth. In fact, part of that was to give them also tools, businesses tools to remain flexible like allowing for carry-on alcohol, which by the way was the most popular thing I've ever done as Governor was allow for that.

And then, of course, we've got the vaccines. And that's something we've been continuing to emphasize with citizens here in Nebraska is the importance of getting vaccines. In fact, the state of Nebraska just released a report last week that showed with our data that if you are unvaccinated and unboosted, you were 46 more times likely to be in the hospital, and if you were just vaccinated but unboosted, that you're 11 times more likely to be in the hospital. And that's part of our campaign of continuing to educate people. And that's been a key part of this throughout the whole thing is communication.

During the height of the pandemic, we had seven press conferences a week, two in Spanish. We translated our materials into multiple languages to be able to reach people. We had, as I mentioned, different groups that we worked with directly, whether it was folks who were bilingual to be able to help get the message out, community leaders, and so forth to really help Nebraskans understand how they can take care of each other and take care of themselves. And so that's been a big part of this is doing the communication.

And now, as the chairman pointed out, we've got Omicron, which is far more transmissible. And certainly as the chairman pointed out, our experience in Nebraska is also that it is not as virulent as the previous strains were. So, for example, even though on January 10 we saw a record amount of testing, over 28,000 tests, we saw that also with the record amount of cases, as I think some of my colleagues here have expressed, we're not seeing that turn into the same number of hospitalizations we would have expected, say, in November 2020.

In fact, we continue to monitor hospital capacity such that we know that, you know, emergency rooms, for example, typically operate at 95 to 97 percent capacity. And in Omaha, our large metropolitan area right now, our emergency rooms are operating about 90 percent capacity. I know Lincoln is a little over 80 percent.

So, again, we continue to focus on that hospital capacity to supply that hospital bed, that ICU bed, or that ventilator to anybody who needs it. We're also seeing from our health officials, who we stay in constant contact with, that, for example, the people who are in our ICU beds tend to be more Deltas—predominantly more Delta. And the folks who do have Omicron and are on, say, a ventilator are staying on those ventilators for a shorter period of time.

So, what are we doing here in the state of Nebraska with regards to this new surge of Omicron? Well, one of the things we're doing is to supplement the Federal administration's testing that they're sending out to everybody. We're also implementing our own at-home testing that includes video links with medical professionals. And then, as I think one of my previous colleagues mentioned, importantly it links back into our health systems so we can track those, should the person agree to do that. We want to make sure that with that at-home testing, we're capturing that data as well. We're also doing something that we did during the pandemic, which is opening up more hospital capacity by finding spaces for people who are in the hospitals but don't need that acute level of care. Maybe they need a skilled nursing level of care, and they don't have a facility right now, or maybe they just need that rehabilitation discharge being home. So, we're looking to be able expand that by about a hundred hospital beds in Omaha, Lincoln, and Grand Island to be able to create more capacity for our hospitals. And then, of course, we're also looking to be able to not only increase the testing through the home kits, but using a vast public health plan with our private partners who are doing testing, to be able to help them be able to find the ability to be able to get the test done and turnaround quickly.

So, I see that I have already run out of time with regard to it. So, Chairman, I'll be respectful of the committee here. But happy to answer any questions. And, again, thank you very much for giving us the opportunity to talk about what we've done here in Nebraska to be able to help keep Nebraskans safe without lockdowns, mask mandates, vaccine passports.

We've asked Nebraskans to do the right thing. We've taking a balanced approach to be able to slow the spread of the virus, protect our hospital capacity, and let Nebraskans live a more normal life. And that's how we're going to continue to manage the pandemic in our state.

Thank you.

Chairman CLYBURN. Thank you very much, Governor. Finally, we will hear from Governor Inslee.

Governor Inslee, you are recognized for five minutes.

Statement of Governor Jay Inslee, State of Washington

Mr. INSLEE. Thank you, Mr. Chairman.

It's a joy to be here. It's a joy to be with my old colleagues. It's a joy to see three members of the 103d Congress. You were rookies, now you're running America, so it's a joy to join you.

You know, our perspective, I think it's interesting, because we had the very first case on January 21, 2020. We had our first death in America, which was on February 29. And we started this with no template. We didn't get to, you know, cadge ideas from Colorado or anywhere else. We were the first. And we made some really early decisions that I think have served us well.

No. 1, we did decide to follow science and the data and our public health experts, and to be very vocal against the profoundly malicious efforts to not spread the truth about this vaccine that had been so damaging.

No. 2, we made a valued decision that saving lives was our first priority, and it should remain unwavering.

And third, we made the decision that the best way we could possibly reopen our economy is to knock down the virus.

Now the question is, did those strategies work? They worked big time. And I want to talk to you about that.

We believe that we saved perhaps 17,000 lives because of following these policies. I want to show you a graph that I think is instructive. If we can put up the COVID graph, if you will, please, on or screens. I look forward to seeing that, if you can get that up for us. I hope that that can come up fairly shortly. Are you guys seeing it, because I'm not.

Here we go. OK. So, we're looking at a graph. On the right, our deaths per 1,000 were about 133. We wish it was zero. But put that in perspective to other states, many of whom have not followed the measures that I just talked about. You'll see the national average is 256. That's in the gray bar. So, our death rate per 100,000 is just about half what the national average is.

But it gets more depressing than that. You look at some of the other states, working up to the left, where the furthest one on the left has almost, you know, three times the death rate. Think about that. And so when you look at this from a national perspective, if the Nation had succeeded the way Washington State has succeeded, perhaps 400,000 people would not have lost their lives. Think about that. That's almost the number of people we lost in World War II.

So, these measures that we have adopted have had profound success in saving lives. And I just want to talk to you about the things we've done that I believe have had success.

Let me start with masks. We believe—thank you, you can put the slide down, I think.

The most successful thing we've done is masks. They have been embraced throughout Washington. There has been very high compliance with some of our mask mandates. They have kept our businesses open. They're now keeping our schools open. And people have embraced it, and I'll tell you why.

People talk about freedom? I think Americans should have freedom not to be infected by their coworker, or infected by their student, their fellow student. That's a freedom. And my state has embraced that concept that has saved lives big time. We've made over 5 million masks just available in the last two weeks. They're readily available and people are using them.

Second issue, vaccinations. We're now at about 80 percent. This is pivotal because 80 percent of the people that are in our hospitals are the unvaccinated. This is a serious disease of the unvaccinated at this moment. And one of the things we've done has been very successful, which is we have increased vaccination rates amongst our state employees, our hospital workers, and our educational community by making it a condition of employment. That has increased our vaccination rate from 50 percent to 96 percent. Twenty- eight thousand people who are employees of mine are now protected who were not protected. And we only lost about three percent of our state employees as a result, and saved massive amount of time off from these folks who otherwise would have been hospitalized.

Look, my DOT had 17,000 days lost due to COVID hospitalizations. We're saving people to keep them on the job. This has worked big time.

We're helping our economy. Now, some folks thought the things we proposed would hurt our economy. If you can put up the economy slide just for a moment. Some folks posited that the things we did of masking and vaccines would hurt our economy. I just want to show you what our economy is doing relative to the rest of the state—country. If you can just put up that economy slide. I hope you can shoot that one up there for us in due time.

This is significant. Our unemployment rate dipped about a percent. Compare this to some other states that took the position that perhaps they weren't willing to take some of these measures. You'll see that we have done very well. The USA average is three percent. Our economy has boomed relative to other places when we have done these things to keep this down.

Brief note on schools. Ninety-six percent, really about four percent of our schools are not in person right now. We've been very successful with our masking requirements. And we reordered our schools to go back to school in person in June, and this has worked very, very well.

Last comment on testing. We have increased our capacity. We do about 500,000 tests a week through our schools. And now we have—or in the next couple of days, we're going to have, I think, a unique ability to get your tests through Amazon. So, you'll be able to go online, and Amazon has helped us distribute these masks. We're moving forward on that.

Last comment of how you can help, besides sending money, which, of course, Governors always do, that's our bottom line. But I would make a note, and I'm following Governor Polis on this, we need nurses, we need mental health treatment in our schools for our kids. This is a big time need right now. I'm proposing a whole bunch in my budget. You can help where you can.

With that, look forward to your questions.

Chairman CLYBURN. Thank you very much, Governor. Thank you so much to all of the witnesses today.

Now each member will have five minutes for questions, and the chair recognizes himself for five minutes.

I have one question for, that I would like a quick response from all of the Governors and the Mayor too, and that is this: Since we've been putting up charts—Governor Inslee you put up a couple of charts—I hope that we can get a chart that I have pertaining to the state of Washington. And this chart showed something that I wanted to bring everybody's attention to. It's clear. And this is from the state of Washington.

Among the unvaccinated, literally the numbers are clear as to what's happening with unvaccinated as opposed to the vaccinated. And that's a big problem for us. Now, though the deaths are less, hospitalizations, not as severe, but the problem is people are getting sick and they're filling up the hospitals. And hospitals are now complaining that it's going to be a problem.

These high hospitalizations are a problem for us. Now I want to know from you, Governor Inslee, why do you believe that the unvaccinated residents in the state of Washington continue to remain unvaccinated? What do you suggest? What can we do to deal with this issue?

And I'm going to come to you next, Governor Ricketts, and the rest of that. I just want to know what you think we can do.

Governor Inslee?

Mr. INSLEE. There we go. Yes. Well, the first thing we can do is make vaccination as easy and convenient as possible. We've done that with our max vaxx sites. We've opened up another one. And it's very important to get people boosted.

Before I leave here, I want to say, look, boosting is everything right now. It is so much more effective than just the first two shots. So, focus on the educational component of that, of letting people know the value of getting boosted.

Second, we can do some of the things for appropriate parts of our community to make this a job requirement. And as you've indicated, this has been very successful saving lives of people who are in the educational community. I believe that if you're a public servant, you shouldn't go around infecting the public. So, we decided our folks would be vaccinated to avoid that and keep you from getting sick so you couldn't work for the state.

And third, in healthcare, obviously, that's been successful as well. But there is an important point I want to talk, if I may, just a moment. I know this is a $64,000 question: Why have about 30 percent of Americans not decided to get the vaccination right now? And I do tell you it is extremely frustrating to me to look at this fact. Of the top reddest counties compared to—areas compared to the top 10 blue areas in the state of Washington, you have a six time higher death rate, six time higher death rate because you're not getting vaccinated amongst people who share more of the red persuasion. And this is an enormous tragedy.

And we have to ask ourselves, why is there such a disparate difference between these two groups of people? And, unfortunately, it is because a lot of folks in the red camp have created an identity that in order to wear the red jacket, you shouldn't be vaccinated. And that is a persistent problem of identity. It's not lack of information. My folks have information coming out their ears.

It's an issue that the Republican Party has created an identity, unfortunately, that has bred a mistrust of science, a mistrust of governmental actions in this regard, and a sense that you can't be a good Republican if you get vaccinated. I think this is a tragedy in our country.

And I urge all my Republican colleagues to resist that. Shoot, I saw the Governor of Florida the other day didn't even want to admit he was boosted. He thought somehow that would make him a bad Republican. This is a tragedy. And it's this issue of identity we've got to get out of our teams and just help our people save their lives.

Chairman CLYBURN. Thank you, Jay.

I believe in equal time. I'm not one of those people who wants to get rid of equal time, so I'm going to give Governor Ricketts equal time. And I ask the indulgence of the ranking member as I do.

Mr. RICKETTS. Well, thank you very much, Mr. Chairman.

You know, as I travel the state of Nebraska and talk to people why they're not vaccinated, the No. 1 thing they tell me is because they don't know who to believe. And I think one of the things that we all need to remember is that typically it takes 10 to 15 years to develop a vaccine. The previous record time to develop a vaccine was four years, and that was the 1960's and that was mumps. And I am very grateful that this only took eight years to develop under Operation Warp Speed—or, sorry, eight months to develop under Operation Warp Speed. But it also hasn't given the public the time to have this information disseminated and to be digested, which normally happens with other vaccines. So, I think that's one thing we've got to keep in mind.

I think we also have to keep in mind that there's been, even from the sources like the CDC, you know, different information coming out. Just start with masks. First, we weren't supposed to get masks for people and then we were supposed to get masks for people and so forth.

So, I think that it is one of those cases where we have to continue to be able to educate people. Again, that's one of the reasons why we released our report last week.

I think also one of the things at this point—you asked what more can we do to get people to get vaccinated. I think that really when it comes down to it, it's going to have to be that friend, family, neighbor, somebody close to the unvaccinated person who makes the case for why they should get vaccinated. I certainly continue to go out and tell people and make the case why they should get vaccinated. As I mentioned, providing the data for vaccinated and boosted versus unvaccinated to people so that they know the risks they're taking by not being vaccinated.

I personally tell people who've been—I've had people who tell me, I got the virus, I don't need to get vaccinated. I'm like, no, you still need to get vaccinated because it will help you build the antibodies to fight a virus in the future. So, we are going to have to engage people.

One of the things we've tried to do here at the state of Nebraska is find local people and run local ads. You know, we—people who have—you know, we recognize within the community, and talk about, for example, how severe COVID was for them, and how it knocked them down and so forth, sent them to the hospital, so that people they can hear locally and know will see that and say, oh, OK, that's a local person. I understand. Maybe I will go get vaccinated.

In fact, I'd say actually just a week or so ago, we had a record date for people who haven't been vaccinated getting their vaccine.

So, I do think that we have to continue to educate people. I think it's got to be local people.

I would disagree with Governor Inslee's characterization that this is a Republican Party thing. I think what we have to do if we really went to get past this is we have to get past the partisanship on this and have to focus on, you know, why are people are not doing it. And in my experience in Nebraska is because people still have to have time to digest this information, and it really needs to be somebody locally telling them, hey, this is something important to help protect your health.

Chairman CLYBURN. Well, I thank you very much. I know my time is up.

I just want to say, as I go to the ranking member for his questions, I've watched over several days ago, as you know, the lead researcher for the Moderna was a relatively young African-American woman who was given credit for having come up with that vaccine. What was interesting to me listening to her when she talked about how quickly they were able to get the final product. They had been working on it for years, working on it for years. They didn't have press conferences every morning saying, we're going into the lab and do some research today. For years, they've been working on this, and they had things all lined up.

So, when they got the information from China and South Africa, they were able to do things rather quickly because they had been working for a decade. And people say it happened too quickly. It did not happen quickly. What happened quickly was the end result.

With that, I yield to the ranking member.

Mr. SCALISE. Thank you for that, Mr. Chairman.

And I know we've got a few of our former colleagues that are testifying.

I'd ask—Cathy McMorris Rodgers, who's the ranking member of the Energy and Commerce Committee, also from the state of Washington, asked if she could have a statement submitted into the record. So, Mr. Chairman, I'd ask unanimous consent if Congresswoman McMorris Rodgers' statement could be entered into the record as well?

Chairman CLYBURN. Without objection, so ordered.

Mr. SCALISE. Thank you.

I'll start with former colleague Jared Polis, Governor Polis. I appreciate you being here. I know I've watched, in your state of Colorado, you've talked about after the vaccine how that's helped alleviate some of the health crisis in Colorado. You had said that, quote: Public health officials don't get to tell people what to wear, meaning face masks; that's just not their job.

I know with your state, you've gotten rid of the mask mandate, no vaccination mandate statewide. How has that worked out in your state and, you know, continued to keep your state going and protect the health of your people?

Mr. POLIS. Yes. This is really a matter—thank you, Representative Scalise—of us having a lot more tools than we had in the early days of the pandemic. In the early days of the pandemic, there was no vaccine. There was not even widespread ability—availability of medical-grade masks. The few masks we had had to be used in the hospital setting. There were not effective treatments. Later on, steroids came, somewhat effective. But nothing like what we have now in terms of the monoclonal, the new drugs coming online.

So, it's a very different situation we were in than early 2020. And so it demands a different kind of response that employs all of the above, right? First and foremost, encouraging people to get vaccinated, all three doses. Incredibly important.

If I looked down for a moment while the others were speaking it was because a friend of mine has COVID. She's in her 70's, and I think she's only alive now because she was able to get vaccinated [inaudible].

Mr. SCALISE. And I know my time's limited. And, yes, we've all seen people who get COVID, as you mentioned, you know, your friend. I know a friend who's vaccinated who got COVID. You know, anybody who suggests that if you get vaccinated, you're not going to get it; only the people unvaccinated pass it on. That's not science, actually; that's misinformation. But I appreciate that.

Let me go to Governor Ricketts because—Governor Ricketts, first, for anybody to suggest that it's a political party spewing anti-vaccination information. Frankly, it was Joe Biden and Kamala Harris as candidates for President and Vice President who tried to put doubt on when Donald Trump was heading up Operation Warp Speed on what might come out of that. But it's not a political party that owns it, even though they did that.

I want to go to success rates. Look, Politico did the report I think you cited in your opening statements. They ranked every single state, all 50 states, on how they faired through COVID. And your state came out No. 1 as the best state to respond. Frankly, I think if we should be hearing from anybody about what to do, some Governors shut everything down. Some Governors have kept things open and mixed results. You've done both. You've kept things open and you've protected your people all combined better than anybody. You kept your schools open, helping those kids, millions of kids across this country whose lives are being destroyed because of that. How did you do it so successfully? What can we replicate with other states who haven't done it as successfully, while keeping everything open?

Mr. RICKETTS. Yes, I think it gets back to, you know, I laid out that plan that we had, that seven-point plan. And it is—a lot of that plan also evolves around communication, just reaching out, as I mentioned, doing it in multiple languages, getting to different groups that would be more at risk, like long our-term care facilities. We had a plan from the University Nebraska Medical Center to address that. Meat processing plants. We had weekly calls for nearly three months with those facilities to talk about best practices, to change the way they were doing things, to slow the spread there.

We worked with our schools on what they could do, helping them all come up with plans for how they could get kids back in classrooms. I really want to credit our teachers who were double- planned sometimes, right, from the kids in the classrooms and the kids who still wanted to be remote.

So, we really—and then, of course, we looked at areas where we had folks who were going to come from a disadvantaged socio-economic background and work with community health centers, for example, to make sure that folks had access to the testing and the contact tracing and the PPE and vaccines when they became available. But it was a lot of communication to be able to get that message out.

And then we focused on things such as, you know, keeping our mortality rate down. According to the Kaiser Family Foundation, we were tied for the seventh lowest mortality rate of any state where people have gotten COVID, you know, among people who got COVID.

We won as best state for kids in classrooms. I think we were No. 6. Politico ranked us No. 4 as far as kids', you know, learning loss. We had almost no learning loss in Nebraska.

And, of course, with regard to, you know, protecting livelihoods, giving people the tools to be able to function in this new environment, giving them flexibility, whether it was waiving licensing restrictions or supervising restrictions or, you know, providing guidance to houses of worship of how they could still have services and so forth.

All those things allow people to have a more normal life. And that's what led—you know, for example, we've got the lowest
only in state history, but in the history of the United States. So, it really was striking this balance among all these things that allowed us to really address this.

And, frankly, it gets back to Nebraskans who, when we communicated out the right thing, they did the right thing. You know, over 90 percent of our seniors are vaccinated. That's where 80 percent of our fatalities come from. So, again, targeting the most at-risk communities is really one of the things that helped us be successful.

Mr. SCALISE. Thanks a lot for that.

Mr. Chairman, appreciate it. I yield back.

Chairman CLYBURN. Thank you, Mr. Scalise.

I'll now yield to Ms. Waters for five minutes of questions.

Ms. WATERS. Thank you very much, Mr. Clyburn. I thank you so much for this hearing. It's so important.

And let me thank all of our witnesses today for the hard work that they're doing to save lives. Our cities and our states with representatives like you have today literally have been doing the kind of work that not only saves lives, but it also helps us to understand what else we need do in order to be of assistance to them.

I am one that understands very thoroughly that resources make a difference to the degree you have the resources that you need to fight the fight, and in this case, it means masks. It means all of the testing materials that are needed. It means the vaccinations. To the degree that they have this, they can continue to do the kind of work that they're doing.

I am so worried, however, that this growing political movement by these anti-vaccine activists and pro-Trump Republicans, it's undermining their work. We find, I'm told, in some of the research that's done, that it is found that there's a huge correlation between belief in misinformation and being unvaccinated. This was said by a woman named Liz Hamel, who heads public opinion research for the Kaiser Family Foundation, a nonpartisan healthcare think tank.

Between conservative media and GOP politicians, many Republican voters are being pummeled with bad science about vaccines almost daily. Kaiser's polling found that 94 percent of Republicans think one or more false statements about COVID–19 and vaccines safely might be true. Over the past eight months, Hamel has watched as Republican vaccination rates have fallen further and further behind the rest of Americans.

While Republicans tracked other groups in terms of vaccination rates earlier this year, Kaiser's research shows that now an unvaccinated person is three times as likely to lean Republican as they are to lean Democrat.

A new analysis by NPR suggests that Republicans are probably dying at a higher rate as a result. A nationwide comparison of 2020 Presidential election results in COVID–19 death rates since vaccines became available to all adults found that counties that voted heavily for Trump had nearly three times the COVID–19 mortality rate of those that went for Joe Biden. Those counties also had far lower vaccination rates. Counties that went heavily for Donald Trump have seen much lower vaccination rates and much higher death rates.

Now, to our witnesses here today, while you talk about some of the things that you're doing, you know, having some Ambassadors, volunteer people going out talking with folks, do you think that you can be more definitive?

For example, you have someone who is advising people—and I'm going to see if I can get his name—to drink their own urine. And so when you have this kind of misinformation that is constantly, you know, bombarding folks, it undermines all the work that you're doing.

Can you get more definitive? Can you describe better? Can you have in your ads, you know, real life information about people who are not vaccinated are dying at a later rate. Can you put that up and out as we should be thinking about how we should do it?

Let me go right to any one of our—Mr. Inslee, since you're from us and you've worked with us, you know what we try and do. What do you think about being tougher, more definitive, and using the words that need to be used in order to dissuade people from not getting vaccinated?

Mr. INSLEE. Well, let me—first, I want to congratulate Governor Ricketts. He's done some good things in Nebraska, congratulate him for some of his successes. But I do think there just is a sad reality we have to recognize, and that is that there has been a profoundly different approach to this whole pandemic, you know, based on whether you're red or blue. That's just the reality.

And when we started this, the defeated President continually belittled the importance of this, said it's going to be over by Easter. And I remember asking him for help early on in this pandemic. He said it wasn't his job to help the states. And now we've got a President I think who's really helping out every time we ask for help. And it started there.

But I just want to suggest that this is a larger problem than just COVID. The virus of deception about our organs of democracy, there's two viruses: one is a virus of COVID and one is falsity. And that falsity is not just about COVID. It's about who won the last election.

Listen, if you have one party telling their Members that you can't trust government enough to even decide who won the last election, it's pretty certain they're not going to trust government when government shares the truth about this virus and the effectiveness of vaccines. And the sad truth is we have one party that has created the big lie certainly about who won the last election and significant mistruths for many—and I'm not counting Governor Ricketts this camp—but many of his colleagues have continued to belittle the effectiveness of these measures. And that's just a sad reality.

Now, how do we change that situation? We try to appeal to the better angels of their nature to knock it off and stop supporting and nominating candidates who want to continue to lie about basic truths in our democracy. That's the infection we have of willing to infect people with falsity. And we saw it on January 6——

Ms. WATERS. Yes.

Mr. INSLEE.—and we saw it every day when I can't get Republicans to get vaccinated. And by the way, in my state—unfortunately, I just have to share you this—in my state, there is a profound difference in the vaccination rates between the red and blue counties in my state. That's just a reality. And I can't get Republicans enough to respond to that. Maybe Governor Ricketts can convince them.

Chairman CLYBURN. Thank you, Governor.

Ms. WATERS. Thank you, Chairman.

Chairman CLYBURN. The gentlelady's time has expired.

Ms. WATERS. Thank you.

Chairman CLYBURN. The chair now recognizes

Mr. Jordan for five minutes.

Mr. JORDAN. Thank you, Mr. Chairman.

It's good to see some of our former colleagues. I want to thank all our witnesses for being here.

I first want to go to what the chairman said in his opening statement a couple hours ago. He attacked Senator Johnson and Representative Gaetz about statements they had made. And then we just heard Governor Inslee say that government shares the truth. That is—I mean, think about what we have been told about this virus that turned out not to be true.

The President of the United States said we have a plan. The President of the United States said we would shut down the virus. Dr. Fauci and CDC and the government said it didn't start in the lab. They all said it wasn't gain-of-function research. They said, we'll never impose a mandate, but they did, so much so, it went to the Supreme Court and the Supreme Court struck it down.

They told us that the vaccinated can't get it. They told us that the vaccinated can't transmit it. They told us there's no such thing as natural immunity. The last thing you want to do is trust what these people have told us, because everything they've told us has turned out to be misleading and not accurate.

Governor Ricketts, are there more people vaccinated now than there were a year ago?

Mr. RICKETTS. Yes, absolutely. As I mentioned, we just had a record day for the number of people who have never been vaccinated to get vaccinated. So, it's a——

Mr. JORDAN. Are there more people who—nationwide, are there more COVID deaths this year than there were last year?

Mr. RICKETTS. You know, I have not tracked the COVID deaths. I heard earlier on a call there were more deaths this year than last year, but I can't tell you. I've been focused on my state. I can't tell you.

Mr. JORDAN. Are there an uptick in cases, as we speak now, nationwide than compared to a year ago?

Mr. RICKETTS. Well, certainly in Nebraska, we've got an uptick in cases, absolutely.

Mr. JORDAN. Yes. There's an uptick everywhere. So, I think the simple question is, how can that be? I mean, if mask mandates and lockdowns work, then why didn't they work? I mean, we've seen all kinds of restrictions placed on the American people, all kinds of limits placed on their freedom. If those things all work, how can we have higher caseloads at a time when there are more people vaccinated and, unfortunately, more people have lost their lives this year than before?

Do you have a mask mandate on schools in your state, Governor Ricketts?

Mr. RICKETTS. No. We've never had a statewide mask mandate ever throughout the pandemic. Different school districts will choose to do mask mandates, but that is the—that is up to the local school districts. We've never done it at the state level.

Mr. JORDAN. You haven't mask mandated businesses in your state.

Mr. RICKETTS. No, we do not.

Mr. JORDAN. Do you have a vaccine passport mandate in your state, as many cities are now imposing on citizens?

Mr. RICKETTS. No, we do not.

Mr. JORDAN. And in your state, by just about any metrics and measure, I looked at some of this prior to the hearing, you've done very well in all kinds—I mean, one of the things I noticed is you've actually had more families move into your state over the time of the pandemic, which cannot be said for New York, New Jersey, California, and D.C., the hardest lockdown states in the country. They've actually seen families and individuals leave their state, move out of their state, and move to states where they actually had freedom. So, you actually went up in people moving to your state. Is that right?

Mr. RICKETTS. Yes, we've certainly got anecdotal evidence to show that there are a lot of people who moved to Nebraska for the quality of life here.

Mr. JORDAN. Quality of life there. That's—I would just call it freedom and quality of life. It's a great state. I've been to your state as many of these other places where people are moving.

When COVID first happened, did you have some regulations you placed on your economy and on your—on the citizens early on like most of the country did when we didn't know a darn thing about this virus? Did you do that?

Mr. RICKETTS. Yes. Absolutely. So, it gets back to what I said earlier about slowing the spread of the virus so we could buildup the capacity and ultimately get the vaccines, all with the goal of protecting our hospital capacity. And as we built up that capacity and got the vaccines, we did not need to have those restrictions in place. So, we've loosened those up significantly, really taking almost all of them off in June.

And then with the staffing emergency, we do have some directed health measures, specifically around hospital capacity and staffing again, releasing the restrictions on occupational licensing and supervision requirements, that sort of thing, to give hospitals more capacity and more flexibility in managing their caseloads.

Mr. JORDAN. Well, I guess maybe one of the questions I asked too is when you—when you did have those restrictions early on in this—during the virus, did you follow, you as the leader of your state, did you follow the restrictions you had in place?

Mr. RICKETTS. Oh, yes, absolutely. I had to quarantine twice. Most recently, I was exposed and had to wear a mask for 10 days.

Mr. JORDAN. Yes. But this is—this is one of the things that dri-—at least the people I talked to in the Fourth District of Ohio, one of the things that drives them crazy is this double standard. I mean, Mayor Bowser, she had a quarantine requirement in place and didn't follow it, because she had to go visit with Joe Biden after the election last year when she left the state and didn't follow. The very requirement she put on her citizens, she wouldn't follow. And time and time again we have seen elected officials, most often they seem to be from the other party, who won't follow the very restrictions they place on the people they're supposed to represent and the people who pay their salary, won't follow the very restrictions they put on those people.

So, it's—I'm glad that you—you did that.

Any idea—last question, Governor Ricketts, any idea how many people work at the CDC?

Mr. RICKETTS. I have no idea how many people work at the CDC. Mr. JORDAN. Ten thousand people, 10,000 people work there. Any idea how many studies they've done on natural immunity at the CDC or, frankly, at the NIH?

Mr. RICKETTS. I'm not aware of any on natural immunity. In fact, I think we're the only major country in the world that does not recognize natural immunity.

Mr. JORDAN. Could you hazard a guess of why the NIH and CDC, with combined over 30,000 employees and an annual budget combined of over $56 billion, why they wouldn't do a study on natural immunity? Any idea? Could you hazard a guess?

Mr. RICKETTS. I have no idea. I can only imagine they just were not told to do so.

Mr. JORDAN. Yes. OK.

With that, Mr. Chairman, I yield back.

Chairman CLYBURN. I thank the gentleman for yielding back. The chair now recognizes Ms. Maloney for five minutes.

Ms. MALONEY. Thank you, Mr. Chairman. And I want to thank you for having this very important hearing.

And it is great to see three of my former colleagues here today. Congratulations on all the good work you're doing.

But I'm going to address my questions to Mayor Bowser. I have a special relationship with D.C., having spent so much time there. I would like to explore, Madam Mayor, how Republican efforts to block D.C.'s statehood could have possibly hampered the District's response to the coronavirus pandemic.

Throughout 2020, as the virus crisis took hold across the District and the country, D.C. residents and businesses received less than half the amount of CARES Act relief funds they would have been entitled to as a state, depriving the District residents of roughly $755 million in pandemic relief for a year. Thankfully, congressional Democrats, including myself and those of us on the Oversight Committee, worked with the Biden administration to retroactively restore this funding through the American Rescue Plan.

But that critical funding came a year late for the residents of the District. D.C. residents pay more in Federal taxes per capita than residents of any other state, and they have been disproportionately impacted by the pandemic and its outsized harm on communities of color.

So, Mayor Bowser, how did the delay in relief funding impact the District's ability to respond to the coronavirus pandemic?

Ms. BOWSER. Well, thank you, Representative Maloney. And thank you for your leadership and all of your support for the District.

And it was a huge distraction, first and foremost, $755 million, three-quarters of a billion dollars is a lot of money for anybody, and it's especially a lot of money for us. For some reason we're yet to figure out, in the CARES Act, our state level funding, which we received for all matters of Federal funding, was limited. And we received $755 million less than we should.

What we did in its place not to hamper our building up our capacity, as you've heard all of the Governors mention, we were able to tap into some of our reserves so that we could continue to advance our response. However, your efforts to get that money restored allowed us to maintain our very critical government operations and the emergency response.

Ms. MALONEY. Thank you.

Now, also D.C.'s lack of statehood creates additional barriers for its pandemic response efforts. For example, Governors in other states, including those with us today, have deployed members of their National Guard to support hospital staff and testing efforts during the recent Omicron surge. But as we know, D.C. does not have full authority over its National Guard and cannot activate them without approval from the Secretary of Defense.

My question, Mayor Bowser, is: How has the lack of statehood created unique hurdles for the District? And how has this undermined your efforts, D.C.'s response, to the coronavirus?

Ms. BOWSER. Thank you, Representative Maloney. It's true that calling the D.C. National Guard is kind of a misnomer. It's really the President's Guard. Unlike all of the 50 states, our Guard is basically under the command of the President of the United States. When we use our Guard, I submit a request to the DOD to get that request met. In years past, that has been pretty pro forma and it's happened quickly. We saw, however, in the last four years, that those requests were delayed, sometimes limited, as with our request for support on January—on the events leading up to January the 6. They're also limited in the fact that we can't change them mid-mission, which, you know, circumstances change, as we saw on January the 6. And the Mayor of the District cannot direct those changes.

There have been proposals. Our Congresswoman has, you know, advanced legislation to change that. It's been supported in the Senate to change that. Unfortunately, that didn't get done this year, but it needs to get done.

Our National Guard, I had called them up to support the coronavirus efforts, and they were very helpful in setting up our testing. We have recently called for them to again to support testing in Omicron.

Ms. MALONEY. Well, also, Madam Mayor, over the recent holidays, Omicron drove cases and hospitalizations to new highs in D.C., one of the epicenters of the latest wave of the virus. And although the District's vaccination campaign has thankfully worked to reduce the rate of severe diseases and death compared to prior waves of the pandemic, our colleagues across the aisle have taken steps in recent weeks to try to impede these efforts to save lives. Republicans have introduced no fewer than five bills in this Congress in an effort to undermine D.C.'s critical work to increase vaccinations among District residents. Madam Mayor, how do these efforts risk endangering your government's response and the health and safety of District residents?

Ms. BOWSER. Well, I think the whole point——

Chairman CLYBURN. Madam Mayor, cut it real short.

Ms. BOWSER. Yes.

I think the whole point of what we've been talking about is the Governors, the chief, and the mayor here know best for our states. And we know best for the District of Columbia what works. We're not all the same. We're urban, we're dense, and we have to have strategies in place that will keep our residents and our city safe. And is that is what we have advanced.

Ms. MALONEY. Thank you.

My time has expired. Thank you. I yield back. Thank you, Mr. Chairman.

Chairman CLYBURN. Thank you very much.

The chair now recognizes Ms. Miller-Meeks for five minutes.

Ms. MILLER-MEEKS. Thank you, Chair Clyburn.

And first off, I want to thank all of our witnesses for testifying before us today and sharing their experiences.

As we all know, the Trump administration under Operation Warp Speed developed three safe and effective vaccines. And as a physician, former director of public health, I can say that it's nothing short of miraculous and it was built on decades of research.

I also want to be abundantly clear, I am fully vaccinated. I've admitted the vaccine in vaccine clinics in all 24 of the counties in my district. And I've encouraged people, persuaded people to be vaccinated, talked with family members of people who ask for guidance in helping their family members to become vaccinated, and will continue to recommend to people to seek guidance from their healthcare providers or physicians about vaccination should they have hesitancy.

However, I don't stand for government mandates and political overreach into the healthcare decisions of individuals. I was pleased to see that the Supreme Court struck down the OSHA mandate, because—in regards to private employers because I felt that that was an unconstitutional overreach of OSHA.

Governor Ricketts, you—can you briefly discuss your states's participation in the lawsuit to stop the mandate?

Mr. RICKETTS. Yes, absolutely. So, again, as I've talked about on this—in the testimony here that, you know, I encouraged people to get the vaccines. And we wanted people to—you know, educate people about doing the right thing, but I also am opposed to the mandates. In fact, as I talk to people, again, who have not been vaccinated yet, one of the really detrimental things that, for example, the mandate on businesses had was there were a number of people who told me—again, this is all anecdotal evidence—but they told me that they were going to get vaccinated but now there is no way they were going to get vaccinated if the Governor was going to be telling them that they had to get vaccinated. So, I think that's one of the downsides when you try to push something.

And, of course, our state, my attorney general and myself, both agreed that trying to use OSHA and really jam, as I think even the chief of staff for the White House, to workaround through this to use OSHA to, you know, push down these vaccines was really outside the law and very detrimental. And it could be used in so many bad ways in the future with an executive branch who then would take this and say, well, I've got a policy I want to enforce. I'm going to find an emergency to declare, and I'm going to tell OSHA to go push my policy through their regulations. That is something that I don't think Republican or Democrat that we want to see the executive branch having that kind of authority to without the—know, going to Congress asking for this kind of authority.

So, that's one of the reasons why our state was one of the states that was taking this to, you know, court because we felt that this was an overreach of the Federal Government and also set a really, really bad precedent for the future. Not—you know, set aside whether or not you think the vaccines are right or not, you're expanding the power of the executive branch hugely by allowing them to go around Congress to enforce this vaccine.

Ms. MILLER-MEEKS. And I thank you for that. And I think what your state and, you know, the other Governors have indicated from their states shows that the Federalist system has worked because different states have different makeups, different rural areas, different population areas, different densities, and so that approach did work.

The Supreme Court in ruling on the OSHA mandate said the right to refuse medical treatment could be overcome when society needs to curb the spread of a contagious epidemic. Vaccines should prevent transmission. As we saw in the Delta variant—and this was CDC, Dr. Walensky, this summer, with the Delta variant and from the Israel study, 45 percent of people would still transmit and have high—high viral loads. And Dr. Walensky said that people infected with Delta is indistinguishable from that—vaxx— unvaccinated people and what the vaccines can't do anymore is present—prevent transmission. We've especially seen this with the Omicron variant, that in the Omicron variant, highly transmissible, less ill.

So what—you know, in mandating a vaccine when there is no longer a public health benefit, i.e., we're not preventing transmission of the virus in the Omicron variant, and we may, in fact, if you read some of the literature on the Danish study that just came out, that there is a negative effect with the vaccine lasting 30 minutes. We may, in fact, create more super variants.

So, I thank you for the job you did, Governor Reynolds [sic]. And our state also did an admiral job. We know in schools that there is increased suicide, increased mental health problems, a detriment to learning, a detriment to not being able to participate, learning loss, school lunches. And I think—can you discuss your decision to allow families to decide what's best for their students and your children in opening schools?

Mr. RICKETTS. Yes. Well, some are like—every state's different and every school district is going to be different, so what we encouraged was I got together with the commissioner of education, who actually is not a cabinet member. He is in a separate elected state Board of Education in Nebraska, so they don't report to me, but we work very closely to come out and set the expectation, in the summer of 2020, that we expected kids to be in classrooms, because we know that it's not just about academic progression but also about, as you mentioned, physical health, mental health, nutrition, socialization. All those things are a benefit. And really worked with our school leaders to—the Department of Education published a book that they worked with us on as well to say here's a roadmap for how you can open up your school.

And so that's what we really did is allowed the school districts to make those decisions, and then, of course, encouraged parents to weigh in with their school boards with regard to that. But that's really how we got to the point where I think one study or one group said that we were the sixth best state for kids in classrooms. As I mentioned, we came out fourth in the Politico study for learning loss. We had very little learning loss in Nebraska, because we did really place an emphasis to try and get those kids back in the classrooms.

Ms. MILLER-MEEKS. Thank you so much, Governor Ricketts.

And I know my time is up. Chair Clyburn, I just know Nebraska and I were [inaudible].

Chairman CLYBURN. I understand. Thank you so much. The chair now recognizes Ms. Vela′zquez for five minutes.

Ms. VELA′ZQUEZ. Thank you, Mr. Chairman.

And it is great to see the many former colleagues on this call. Thank you so much for the great work that you're doing in your respective states.

I would like to ask my first question to Governor Pierluisi. You announced that the American Rescue Plan funding will be used to invest in essential workers and domestic development initiatives. How impactful was this funding for these purposes? And can you please provide specific examples of how your office allocated and prioritized the disbursement of these funds?

Mr. RICKETTS. Yes. So, specifically when it comes to the American Rescue Plan Act—I think this question was addressed to me. Is that right?

Ms. VELA′ZQUEZ. Governor, I relayed my question to Governor Pierluisi from Puerto Rico.

Mr. RICKETTS. Oh, I'm sorry. My apologies.

Ms. VELA´ZQUEZ. OK.

Mr. PIERLUISI. I'll start, and if you want to followup, it'll be fine with me. I'll try to be brief.

It is great to see Congresswoman Vela´zquez participating at this hearing. She was born and raised in Puerto Rico, and she knows the challenges we face, as well as anybody in Puerto Rico.

Actually, the American Rescue Plan has been a blessing for us. We used it, for example, premium pay, hazard pay for workers, essential workers who were out there in the middle of this pandemic last year. I'm talking about, of course, the hospitals, the clinics, but also even restaurants, the entertainment industry, first responders and so on. All workers who were doing in—rendering in-person services while being exposed to this virus deserved this premium pay or hazard pay, and we did it.

We are now doing it still, because this Omicron variant has hit us quite hard. Puerto Rico did so well last year. We had mandates. We had business restrictions and capacity restrictions on businesses at various times during the year. Yet our economy grew, because we were a safe destination for doing business and for visiting us as tourists and so on.

Yet I have to admit, this has been a rough start this year, because the Omicron variant, as has been mentioned before, is very transmissible. And we're seeing—we've just seen case counts that— record case counts, record hospitalization rates. Finally now, it's starting to come down. But I just decided recently to give yet another premium pay to clinic workers at our hospitals and clinics, because we were lucky, Congresswoman, last year, our hospitals were never compromised. But this year, they're quite congested with COVID patients.

Last, I'll just say very quickly——

Ms. VELA´ZQUEZ. Governor?

Mr. PIERLUISI. I'll keep quiet and I'll let you——

Ms. VELA´ZQUEZ. I just have another question and my time is limited.

Mr. PIERLUISI. I know. I know.

Ms. VELA´ZQUEZ. [Inaudible] You know, for the members of the committee to see how important the American Rescue Plan and the impact, the positive impact that it has played in Puerto Rico. And imagine where Puerto Rico would have been today if it had not been for the fact that the Trump—during the Trump year, he withheld disaster relief money appropriated by the Congress of the United States.

Governor, Puerto Rico established also the local Earned Income Tax Credit in 2019. And the American Rescue Plan provided a $600 million supplement for the program. Can you please expand on how the supplemental funding for Puerto Rico's EITC will help strengthen its labor market and help reduce poverty?

Mr. PIERLUISI. Yes. That's the best anti-poverty program in the states. And we've never had a comparable program in Puerto Rico because of our limited resources. We never had access to the EITC. So, what Congress did, and it's great, Congress is basically funding now 75 percent of our local version of the EITC. This is going to give our workers up to about $6,500, up to that amount, as an incentive to join the labor force, to increase our labor participation rate, which has always lagged the one you have in the U.S. mainland.

So, it's going to start this April. When we file tax returns in Puerto Rico, our taxpayers will start getting this for the first time. We also, as part of the American Rescue Plan, got fully included in the child tax credit program. Because, believe it or not, only families with three children or more had access to the child tax credits. Now, all families will. And that's another great help from the American Rescue Plan.

And so what I'll say to just close is that—and I was kind of mentioning it before, the booster is so important. One thing we did in Puerto Rico, Congresswoman Vela´zquez, is that science and medicine have been driving our government decisions. I have been relying on the medical and scientific community in Puerto Rico for my decisions. And that has allowed us to keep politics out of the way. You know that we're very passionate about our politics in Puerto Rico. But since my decisions have been driven by science and medicine, that's why we've had a lot of support from the public at large, from the political class at large. And if I have any recommendation or suggestion for the mainland would be that one.

Ms. VELA´ZQUEZ. Congressman—Governor, I went to Puerto Rico. I spent two weeks for the holidays. I didn't get Omicron. I came back to the United States. I went to Washington, DC, and I came back with Omicron here. So, even after being fully vaccinated.

So, thank you so much for the work that you are doing. I yield back.

Chairman CLYBURN. Thank you very much.

Thank you, Ms. Vela´zquez.

I don't see Ms. Malliotakis. Has she come back?

The chair now recognizes Mr. Foster for five minutes.

Mr. FOSTER. Thank you, Mr. Chair. And thank you to our witnesses.

You know, as a scientist, I find it sort of—well, I had a number of things that I was tempted to react to, but I found it absolutely remarkable to hear one of my colleagues claim that there was no public health benefit of vaccines.

You know, also, I'd like to point out that there's a pretty big difference between absolutely preventing transmission, which, of course, no vaccine ever does, compared to reducing transmission, which they unquestionably do. And I think that the—the fundamental reason why we seem to be talking back and forth past each other is that—is the question of whether or not a government of a country has a right to ask its citizens to take even a small risk or inconvenience for the greater good of its citizens, or whether this is simply viewed as an outrageous intrusion on individual freedom. You know, my draft number was 321. And so—and Hanoi fell in 1973. And I—my number would have come up in 1974, so I was never asked to serve. But I had long discussions with my dad. I would have served. And when the—the soldiers who got drafted for World War II, they did not get to say, my body, my choice. You know, they were asked to take a reas-—a significant risk to fight the Nazis. They were not allowed to say, well, I'm going to wait for more scientific data to see if it is safe to fight the Nazis or not.

They were asked to take—you know, take a risk and to do something for their country to keep their fellow citizens safe. And it seems as though, frankly, today's Republican Party has raised individual, not freedom, but selfishness to a level that it would be inconceivable to the greatest generation.

Anyway, so I just—maybe I can see if this—I had a question actually for Governor Inslee. When you were talking about what you viewed as the partisan tilt and you're seeing it even in the death rates in different—do you think that this is to the extent that it may actually have electoral implications downstream?

Mr. INSLEE. I'm sorry, Bill. I lost the last part of your question. Mr. FOSTER. Do you think that when you look at the differential death rates in the counties, depending on the partisan lean of the counties, do you think this is large enough to have maybe differential, you know, effects on elections downstream when you just look at very close elections? That'd be an interesting analysis to do.

Mr. INSLEE. Well, here's the tragedy of this, and I do believe it is a tragedy. We have a disproportionate number of members of the Republican Party dying in my state. Now, one would think, if you're Republican, you'd really want to be aggressive to prevent losing your people. But we hear voices like Congressman Jordan's, who are continuing to spread disinformation, which is causing health jeopardizing to his people that are in his party. That's a real tragedy.

And then—and when other colleagues, frankly, like Governor Ricketts, who will stand up and try to share valid scientific information, people don't trust them because the members of that party has been telling people for 10 years, don't trust the government. So, that's the situation we're in.

What are the electoral consequences? I'm not sure that's relevant to this particular discussion, but we have to try and save everybody's life here. That's what I'm for.

Mr. FOSTER. Yes. OK. Let's see, there's been also some mention of the parts of the response that were Federalized, the part that were left to the states. Do any of you have any comments on things that the Federal Government should have taken a bigger role in, just particularly in relation to collecting data? Governor Polis?

Mr. POLIS. First of all, I think, you know, many of my fellow Governors, including myself, when the Federal Government can do it well, we welcome them to do it. And that's why I'm glad you're offering testing. We've been doing that for a couple months. We're glad somebody—once we see the Federal Government can do it right, we're happy to stop doing and fold that in. Same with masks. The FEMA crews have been indispensable. Our state's used them during surges. The National Guard has been indispensable. We've used that during our surges. So, there have been key components where I just don't know where we would be at. It would be—not only would it have been much more fatal to members of the public in many states; it also would have been much more devastating to the economy without all those areas of Federal support.

Mr. FOSTER. Yes. Governor? Yes.

Mr. INSLEE. One of the things that is really important in the healthcare system is to have a robust scale of opportunities in the long-term care system. That's the one thing I might suggest we can certainly use more dollars for. Because if you don't have enough places in your long-term care facility, you can't discharge people from your hospital. We're experiencing that problem, so we've been building up our long-term care facility.

But help from Congress to get more long-term care facility opportunities for people, this is pivotal for the healthcare hospital access that we now have shortages of.

Mr. FOSTER. OK. There appears—OK. Quickly, my time has actually expired.

Ms. BOWSER. I just wanted to say quickly, I think the Federal Government getting income in people's hands——

Chairman CLYBURN. Madam Mayor, I'm sorry, the time has expired.

Ms. BOWSER. OK.

Chairman CLYBURN. The chair now recognizes Mr. Raskin for five minutes.

Mr. RASKIN. Thank you, Mr. Chairman, and thanks for conducting this very important hearing.

One of the things we've learned during this grim period in our history is that propaganda works on a lot of people. So, misinformation and disinformation are actually undermining the public health. They promote vaccine hesitancy, they generate social discord, they've destroyed the cohesiveness of our public health efforts. And yet to this day, Members of Congress are spreading anti-public health propaganda.

Let's take a look at some of the examples, if you'd be kind enough to put it up on the screen.

Last month, Representative Gaetz said that, quote: The best vaccine we've found is Mother Nature's vaccine. It's contracting the virus.

Well, this is false and dangerous. The best vaccine we have is a vaccine. Yesterday, the CDC published a study which found that vaccination remains the safest strategy for averting COVID–19 infection, hospitalization, and death. So, his statement is like saying the best vaccine for polio or the German measles is contracting the disease.

Representative Boebert said: Biden has deployed his Needle Nazis to Mesa County.

This is a dangerous lie. It equates state, local, and Federal public health efforts with history's worst fascist dictatorship, a regime responsible for genocidal violence against millions of people. The analogy is an affront to millions of doctors, nurses, and medical personnel, and government workers on the front lines of the struggle to protect us against COVID. And it's an insult to the memory of millions of people slaughtered by the Nazis.

Representative Marjorie Taylor Greene told her supporters, quote: Biden is going to homes to push shots. Just say no.

This kind of propaganda and anti-public health advocacy has created dramatically higher vaccine hesitancy among Republicans than Democrats, and even contributed, as we heard from Governor Inslee, to the disproportionate rates of COVID–19 deaths among Republicans.

And, finally, as the Omicron variant was spreading, the House Judiciary Committee Republicans amplified false insinuations about the effectiveness of booster shots, tweeting: If the booster shots work, why don't they work?

These are just a handful of numerous examples of politicians spreading dangerous misinformation and confusion.

Governor Polis, do you think that false statements like these have undermined vaccination efforts in your state? What have you done to combat them?

Mr. POLIS. Look, I think that everybody should look at the data and make factual statements. Obviously, we have free speech in our country, but we've seen the danger in the tunnels of misinformation that people will go down, spread through, often through social media; sometimes amplified by people in positions of power and authority.

I hope that everybody takes a hard look at the data and uses whatever soapbox they have, however large or small, to really use a fact-based approach to save lives and move past this pandemic. Mr. RASKIN. And, Mayor Bowser, what would you say to fellow elected officials who continue to spread propaganda that discourages Americans from getting vaccinated or from wearing masks? You got to unmute.

Ms. BOWSER. I think it's especially problematic, Congressman, because they themselves have been vaccinated and boosted and are enjoying the benefits of those vaccines. And they know better. And they also, probably more than most of their constituents, know of people who have suffered and died because of this virus.

Nobody should die in our hospitals attached to a ventilator and have to say goodbye to their families when there is a safe and effective vaccine. And we all need to be saying that.

We've heard it said that the vaccine should stop—public health has always said that the vaccine was effective against serious illness, in hospitalization, in death. That has always been the promise of the vaccine, and it is working.

Mr. RASKIN. Thank you.

Governor Inslee, about 75 percent of coronavirus deaths in your state since February 2021 have been among unvaccinated people. And a study conducted last year found that the highest rates of coronavirus death in Washington State were concentrated in the 15 most Republican counties, which is an alarming statistic.

How do you account for this dramatic divide, and what does it tell you about what we need to do?

Mr. INSLEE. Well, No. 1, you mentioned at the outset that propaganda works. Propaganda worked, you know, in the forties, but it works a hundred times more now because of the internet and the algorithms that we have and the ability of the internet to spread a lie. If a lie went 25 miles an hour two decades ago, it goes 250 miles an hour now. And we have seen the impact of that. Just some of the quotes you showed up are certain somebody made egregious things.

But, listen, we have a guy who's been appointed by the Republican Party to sit on the Subcommittee on the Coronavirus Crisis, Congressman Jordan. He's been given by the Republican Party a soapbox to talk about this, and he comes before this committee and spends his five minutes basically saying, you shouldn't trust science. You shouldn't trust the CDC. You shouldn't trust people who tell you vaccine works. And that's what the Republican Party put up as their spokesperson.

We need the Republican Party to take some responsibility here and not put their Members, who are spreading this dangerous filth, to America. And I'm urging all Republicans in good faith to do that.

Mr. RASKIN. Thank you.

And, Mr. Chairman, we've got to stop inflaming people's misunderstandings with propaganda, with conspiracy theory. Let's invest in the health of all Americans.

Thank you for this hearing, and I yield back.

Chairman CLYBURN. Thank you, Mr. Raskin.

The chair recognizes Mr. Krishnamoorthi for five minutes.

Mr. KRISHNAMOORTHI. Thank you, Mr. Chair.

Governor Ricketts, you've been vaccinated, correct?

Mr. RICKETTS. Yes, I've been vaccinated and boosted.

Mr. KRISHNAMOORTHI. Excellent. And I presume that the reason that you were vaccinated and boosted is because you believe in the vaccines, right?

Mr. RICKETTS. That is correct.

Mr. KRISHNAMOORTHI. Now, President Trump recently said, according to The Hill, that elected officials and politicians should disclose that they received a vaccine and booster. And I agree with that sentiment too. And I'm glad that you've publicly stated your vaccination status.

I want to turn to another subject. On June 18, 2020, according to the Omaha Herald World, you told local government officials that they won't get Federal coronavirus relief funding if they require individuals to wear face masks in government buildings.

Now, Omaha, the capital—I'm sorry. Omaha, the largest city in Nebraska, has a mask mandate, including in buildings, and it renewed that mask mandate last Wednesday.

Have you withheld any coronavirus Federal funding from Omaha?

Mr. RICKETTS. So, with regard to that, specifically, actually, Omaha let their mask mandate that passed by city ordinance expire. The county health official has tried to implement a mask mandate illegally, and we're actually going to court over this one.

Mr. KRISHNAMOORTHI. But have you withheld any coronavirus funding from either the county or the city?

Mr. RICKETTS. No, I have not.

Mr. KRISHNAMOORTHI. OK. And how about Nebraska Medicine? Both Nebraska Medicine and the University of Nebraska Medical Center both have mask mandates. Have you withheld any Federal coronavirus funding from either of those two entities?

Mr. RICKETTS. No. And getting back to Omaha as well, the difference in the Omaha one that they did, they also exempted government services from the mask mandate as well. So, again, they were compliant with what I asked, which is don't prohibit people from getting government services because of the mask mandate.

Mr. KRISHNAMOORTHI. No. But in your pronouncement, you said wearing a mask in a Federal Government—I'm sorry—in a government building would be enough to trigger your not giving them relief funding that was provided to you by the Federal Government. Now, has that——

Mr. RICKETTS. Right.

[Crosstalk]

Mr. KRISHNAMOORTHI. Has there been any entity—has there been any entity in Nebraska that did not receive Federal coronavirus relief funding because of your policy that you put in place?

Mr. RICKETTS. No.

Mr. KRISHNAMOORTHI. OK. So, that was just political rhetoric. I get it. Now, in——

Mr. RICKETTS. No. It was because they—no, it wasn't political rhetoric——

Mr. KRISHNAMOORTHI [continuing]. response to the——

Mr. RICKETTS.—the government services, was what I requested. Mr. KRISHNAMOORTHI. In response to the President's vaccine mandate—let me repeat it. A tweet that you put out on September 10, 2021, at 11:10 a.m., you said—in response to the President's mandate, you said: Vaccine mandate. President Biden has forgotten we live in America, quote/unquote.

Quote: He thinks we live in the Soviet Union.

Now, Governor Ricketts, I just want to ask you this question: You don't really believe that President Biden has forgotten we live in America, do you?

Mr. RICKETTS. No. I believe that he forgot that the Federal—the executive branch does not have the authority to issue that——

Mr. KRISHNAMOORTHI. No. I'm just asking you——

Mr. RICKETTS.—which is consistent with what happens in an authoritarian regime.

Mr. KRISHNAMOORTHI [continuing]. you don't believe—you talked about a lot of heated political rhetoric. You don't stand by those statements that you made in that tweet, do you?

Mr. RICKETTS. The point of the tweet was to say that the executive branch does not have the authority to issue a vaccine mandate such as he was doing, similar to what happens in authoritarian——

Mr. KRISHNAMOORTHI. I'm just reading your tweet, Governor,

and you said: He thinks we live in the Soviet Union.

That's what you said in that tweet. You don't really believe that he thinks we live in the Soviet Union, do you?

Mr. RICKETTS. As we all know on this, we've heard plenty of it today, there's plenty of political rhetoric to go by.

Mr. KRISHNAMOORTHI. And you are one of the primary sources of this heated political rhetoric.

Now, sir, you are against government-mandated vaccine mandates, correct?

Mr. RICKETTS. That is correct.

Mr. KRISHNAMOORTHI. And you are also against employer-mandated vaccines?

Mr. RICKETTS. No. Actually, I believe employers have the ability to do that, but I discourage it.

Mr. KRISHNAMOORTHI. You discourage it.

Now, sir, you and I share something in common. We are Cubs fans. Did you know that?

Mr. RICKETTS. I did not know that. Thank you for being a fan. Mr. KRISHNAMOORTHI. And you are a part owner of the Chicago Cubs. Isn't that right?

Mr. RICKETTS. Well, no, not me personally, but a family trust, yes.

Mr. KRISHNAMOORTHI. I understand a family trust owns the Chicago Cubs that you benefit from. Now, you know that the Chicago Cubs have mandated vaccines for their employees, right?

Mr. RICKETTS. Actually, I'm no longer a part of the management of the Cubs, so I was not aware that they had actually mandated vaccines. But as I mentioned before.

Mr. KRISHNAMOORTHI. Well, hold on. Hold on a second. Hold on a second, Governor. The Ricketts family owns the Chicago Cubs. You benefit from the ownership of the Chicago Cubs. The Chicago Cubs requires vaccines and they require masks indoors. I know. I'm a lifelong Cubs fan, and my friends and family all know that you wear a mask when you go to a Chicago Cubs-owned facility, a Ricketts-owned facility.

Thank you, and I yield back.

Chairman CLYBURN. I thank the gentleman for yielding back.

Unless I have missed someone, I think that all attendees have asked their questions, and we've come to the closing.

And I don't see the ranking member. If he's here, I'm going to yield to him. I don't see him.

So, let me thank all of the witnesses for being here today.

And before we close, I want to enter into the record the letters to the committee which were received from Governor Kate Brown of Oregon and Governor Kathy Hochul of New York. I ask unanimous consent that these letters be entered into the official hearing record. So ordered.

Chairman CLYBURN. I want to once again thank Governor Inslee, Governor Polis, Governor Pierluisi, Governor Ricketts, and Mayor Bowser for testifying before the select subcommittee today. We appreciate your insight, your expertise, and your advice on how Governors are responding to the Omicron variant.

I applaud the Biden-Harris administration for its leadership in responding to the Omicron variant and working hand-in-hand with states to support their pandemic response efforts. Among other steps, the Biden-Harris administration has worked with our states to add 10,000 more vaccinationsites, to open additional testing sites, to deploy medical personnel, to help healthcare providers, to order and administer millions more doses of coronavirus treatments, and to make available hundreds of millions of high-quality N95 masks and rapid at-home tests to Americans for free, starting later this month. We are in a better position today than we were a year ago.

As this chart shows, the Biden administration has increased the number of daily tests performed from 1.7 million per day in January 2021 to more than

11.7 million per day in January 2022, a number that is expected to continue rising.

The Biden administration has increased the number of free testing sites around the country eightfold, and worked with the private sector to get 375 million at-home rapid tests on the market this month when there will be zero available just a year ago.

The Biden administration has presided over a historic vaccination campaign that administered more than 500 million vaccines and booster doses over the last year, helping get more than 73 million of adults fully vaccinated.

Our vaccines remain the most powerful tools we have to fight all variants of the coronavirus. Vaccines are free and readily available at more than 90,000 convenient locations across the country.

I encourage everyone to get vaccinated immediately and get their boosters as soon as they are eligible.

All of these steps have helped to reopen more than 95 percent of schools and our economy safely, and will remain critical to our effort to quickly and decisively combat the Omicron variant.

I look forward to working together with leaders at all levels, including and especially today's witnesses, as we continue this progress.

With that, without objection, all members will have five legislative days within which to submit additional written questions for the witnesses to the chair which will be forwarded to the witnesses for their response.

This hearing is adjourned.

[Whereupon, at 5:26 p.m., the subcommittee was adjourned.]

Chapter 8

Science Brief: Omicron (B.1.1.529) Variant*

Centers for Disease Control and Prevention

On November 24, 2021, South Africa reported the identification of a new SARS-CoV-2 variant, B.1.1.529, to the World Health Organization (WHO). B.1.1.529 was first detected in specimens collected on November 11, 2021 in Botswana and on November 14, 2021 in South Africa. South Africa has since detected B.1.1.529 in specimens collected on November 8, 2021. On December 1, 2021, the first case attributed to B.1.1.529 was reported in the United States in a person who returned from travel to South Africa. A second case was reported on December 2, 2021 in a person with no international travel history who also attended a convention in the days preceding symptom onset. The Omicron variant has also been detected in travel- related cases in several European countries, as well as Australia, Brazil, Canada, Hong Kong, Israel, Japan, Nigeria, Norway, Sweden, and the United Kingdom. A few countries, including the United States, have reported cases in individuals without travel history to southern Africa.

On November 25, 2021, the United Kingdom Health Security Agency designated B.1.1.529 as a Variant Under Monitoring (VUI-21-NOV-01).[1] On November 26, 2021, the Technical Advisory Group on SARS-CoV-2 Virus Evolution (TAG-VE)[2] convened to assess B.1.1.529. The TAG-VE advised

* This is an edited, reformatted and augmented version of CDC- Centers for Disease Control and Prevention Publication, updated December 2, 2021.

[1] SARS-CoV-2 variants of concern and variants under investigation (publishing.service.gov.uk)

[2] WHO. Terms of Reference for the Technical Advisory Group on SARS-CoV-2 Virus Evolution (TAG-VE) (www.who.int.)

In: A Closer Look at the COVID-19 Variants
Editor: Richard D. Hylton
ISBN: 979-8-88697-170-5

WHO that this variant should be designated as a Variant of Concern (VOC), and WHO designated B.1.1.529 as a VOC named Omicron.[3]

The WHO classification as a VOC was based on epidemiological data indicating an increase in infections in South Africa in recent weeks that coincided with detection of Omicron. Omicron has many concerning spike protein substitutions, some of which are known from other variants to be associated with reduced susceptibility to available monoclonal antibody therapeutics or reduced neutralization by convalescent and vaccinee sera. The European Center for Disease Prevention and Control also classified this variant as a VOC due to concerns "regarding immune escape and potentially increased transmissibility compared to the Delta variant."[4]

The SARS-CoV-2 Interagency Group (SIG), established by the U.S. Department of Health and Human Services, is responsible for variant classifications in the United States.[i] The SIG meets regularly to evaluate the risk posed by SARS-CoV-2 variants circulating in the United States and globally and to make recommendations about the classification of variants. On November 30, 2021, the SIG made the decision to classify the Omicron variant as a Variant of Concern (VOC). This decision is based on a number of factors, including, detection of cases attributed to Omicron in multiple countries, including among those without travel history, transmission and replacement of Delta as the predominant variant in South Africa, the number and locations of substitutions in the spike protein, and available data for other variants with fewer substitutions in the spike protein indicating a reduction in neutralization by vaccinee and convalescent sera and certain monoclonal antibody treatments.

There are two variants classified as a VOC by the United States: Omicron and Delta. As of December 2, 2021, two confirmed cases attributed to the Omicron variant have been detected in the United States and additional possible Omicron cases are being investigated. Delta continues to be the predominant circulating variant. On August 26, 2021, CDC published information on What We Know About the Delta Variant. Importantly, nearly

---

[3] Classification of Omicron (B.1.1.529): SARS-CoV-2 Variant of Concern (who.int).

[4] Threat Assessment Brief: Implications of the emergence and spread of the SARS-CoV-2 B.1.1. 529 variant of concern (Omicron) for the EU/EEA (europa.eu).

[i] The SIG includes representatives from the Centers for Disease Control and Prevention (CDC), National Institutes of Health (NIH), Food and Drug Administration (FDA), Biomedical Advanced Research and Development Authority (BARDA), and Department of Defense (DoD). This interagency group is focused on the rapid characterization of emerging variants and actively monitors their potential impact on critical SARS-CoV-2 countermeasures, including vaccines, therapeutics, and diagnostics.

all lineages designated as Delta remain susceptible to available monoclonal antibody therapeutics, and vaccines continue to be highly effective against severe illness, hospitalization, and death among people infected with the Delta variant.

Omicron (B.1.1.529) Characteristics

- *WHO Label:* Omicron
- *Pango Lineage:* B.1.1.529
- *Nextstrain clade:* 21K

The spike protein of the Omicron variant is characterized by at least 30 amino acid substitutions, three small deletions, and one small insertion. Notably, 15 of the 30 amino acid substitutions are in the receptor binding domain (RBD). There are also a number of changes and deletions in other genomic regions.

  - *Key Amino Acid Substitutions in Spike Protein (RBD substitutions in bold type):* A67V, del69-70, T95I, del142-144, Y145D, del211, L212I, ins214EPE, **G339D, S371L, S373P, S375F, K417N, N440K, G446S, S477N, T478K, E484A, Q493R, G496S, Q498R, N501Y, Y505H,** T547K, D614G, H655Y, N679K, P681H, N764K, D796Y, N856K, Q954H, N969K, L981F

- *Transmissibility:* Currently, it is unknown how efficiently the Omicron variant can spread from person to person. The replacement of Delta by Omicron as the predominant variant in South Africa raises concerns that the Omicron variant may be more transmissible than Delta, but due to the low number of cases in South Africa when Omicron emerged, it is unclear if this variant is more transmissible than the Delta variant. Further, the relatively small number of cases documented to date makes it difficult to estimate transmissibility. Analysis of the changes in the spike protein indicate that the Omicron variant is likely to have increased transmission compared to the original SARS-CoV-2 virus, but it is difficult to infer if it is more transmissible than Delta.

- N501Y increases binding to the ACE2 receptor, which could increase transmission, and the combination of N501Y and Q498R may increase binding affinity even more; however, other substitutions in the Omicron spike protein are expected to decrease binding to ACE2. As such, receptor binding affinity needs to be assessed using the full spectrum of spike protein substitutions found in the Omicron variant.
- H655Y is proximal to the furin cleavage site and may increase spike cleavage, which could aid transmission.
- N679K is proximal to and adds to the polybasic nature of the furin cleavage site, which may also increase spike cleavage and could aid transmission.
- P681H has been shown to enhance spike cleavage, which could aid transmission. This mutation is found in Alpha and an alternate mutation at this position (P681R) is found in Delta.

- *Disease Severity:* Currently, it is unclear if infection with the Omicron variant is associated with more severe disease. Due to the small number of cases attributed to the Omicron variant, assessment of disease severity is difficult. Preliminary information from South Africa indicates that there are no unusual symptoms associated with Omicron variant infection, and as with other variants, some patients are asymptomatic.[5]
- *Impact on Vaccine-Induced Immunity or Immunity from Previous Infection:* Currently, there are no data available to assess the ability of sera from vaccinated persons or those with previous SARS-CoV-2 infection to neutralize the Omicron variant. However, the U.S. Government SIG and global public health partners are working to generate these data in laboratory settings and will also continue to monitor epidemiological and clinical indicators.
  The spike protein is the primary target of vaccine-induced immunity. The Omicron variant contains more changes in the spike protein than have been observed in other variants, including 15 in the RBD. Based on the number of substitutions, the location of these substitutions, and data from other variants with similar spike protein substitutions, significant reductions in neutralizing activity of sera from vaccinated or previously

[5] Frequently asked questions for the B.1.1.529 mutated SARS-CoV-2 lineage in South Africa – NICD.

infected individuals, which may indicate reduced protection from infection, are anticipated.
Laboratory and epidemiological studies are needed to assess the impact of the Omicron variant on vaccine effectiveness and breakthrough infections, including in individuals who have received booster doses. However, vaccination is anticipated to continue to offer protection against hospitalization and death, and vaccines continue to play a critical role in controlling the COVID-19 pandemic.

- *Impact on Monoclonal Antibody Treatments:* Currently, there are no virus-specific data available to assess whether monoclonal antibody treatments will retain efficacy against the Omicron variant. Based on data from other variants with significantly fewer changes in the RBD, the expectation is that the Omicron variant will remain susceptible to some monoclonal antibody treatments, while others may have less potency.
Mutations within the RBD are most relevant for monoclonal antibody therapeutics available under Emergency Use Authorization (EUA). Currently, there are three monoclonal antibody treatments with EUA: Sotrovimab, Bamlanivimab and Etesevimab, and REGEN-COV.
The following table shows data only for single RBD substitutions that are within the binding site of the indicated monoclonal antibody. However, mutations in the monoclonal antibody binding site do not always result in a loss of binding or neutralization. Importantly, data are needed with the full spectrum of spike protein changes to understand the impact on available monoclonal antibody therapeutics. As data becomes available, the Department of Health and Human Services will rapidly communicate changes in treatment guidance to public health departments and health care providers, as appropriate.

Data in the following table shows data available on the NCATS OpenData Portal[6] that has been tested against a viral variant containing only a single amino acid substitution from a wild-type SARS-CoV-2 in an in vitro neutralization assay.

---

[6] NCATS OpenData Portal: https://opendata.ncats.nih.gov/variant/activity/singlemutationvariant.

In vitro therapeutic activity of single RBD substitutions found in Omicron¥

RBD Substitution	Eli Lilly – Bamlanivimab	Eli Lilly – Etesevimab	Regeneron-Imdevimab	Regeneron – Casirivimab	GSK/VIR-Sotrovimab
G339D					1.18*
S371L					
S373P	No data available				
S375F					
K417N	0.12* 0.367*	>1,000* 381.6*	0.0789* 0.25* 1.2* 1.35*	4.3* 5.67* 7* (7) 13.1* 48.74*	
N440K	No data available		95.63* (28)	1*	0.48*
G446S			No data available		
S477N		0.5*	2.28*	0.91* 2.85*	
T478K	1.25 *	0.231*	0.571*	0.5*	
E484A	No data available			No data available	
Q493R	(100)	No data available	(5)	(70)	
G496S	No data available				
Q498R			No data available	No data available	
N501Y	1* 1.13* (5)	1.65* 2.6* 2.9* (5)	0.1* 0.2* 0.5* 0.62* 0.75* 0.77* 0.95* (2)	0.5* 0.67* 0.9* 0.96* 1* 1.4* 1.64* (2)	
Y505H		No data available			

¥ data as of December 1, 2021.

( ) denotes data from FDA EUA Fact Sheets.

* denotes data from a publication; references below[7,8,9,10,11,12,13,14,15]

Black shaded cells indicate that the substitution is not located in the monoclonal antibody epitope binding region.

- *Impact on Diagnostics:* For the most up to date information and guidance on diagnostic assays, which will be updated to reflect the impact of the Omicron variant, please refer to the U.S. Food and Drug Administration web page on SARS-CoV-2 Viral Mutations: Impact on COVID-19 Tests.
  - The CDC 2019-Novel Coronavirus (2019-nCoV) Real-Time RT-PCR Diagnostic Panel and the Multiplex Assay for Flu and SARS-CoV-2 are expected to detect the Omicron variant.
  - The Thermo Fisher TaqPath COVID-19 Combo Kit (3 total targets) has significantly reduced S-gene target sensitivity due to the deletion at H69 and V70 in the B.1.1.529 (Omicron) spike protein. Specimens being tested using the TaqPath COVID-19 Combo Kit that yield an S gene target failure (SGTF) *could* be Omicron. Importantly, any possible Omicron specimen must be confirmed by sequencing. Since the TaqPath COVID-19 Combo Kit is designed to detect multiple genetic targets, the overall test sensitivity should not be impacted.[16]

Scientists are working to learn more about the Omicron variant to better understand how easily it might be transmitted and the effectiveness of currently authorized or approved medical countermeasures, such as vaccines, therapeutics, and diagnostic tests, against this variant. New information about

---

[7] The dual function monoclonal antibodies VIR-7831 and VIR-7832 demonstrate potent in vitro and in vivo activity against SARS-CoV-2 | *bioRxiv*.

[8] Antibody resistance of SARS-CoV-2 variants B.1.351 and B.1.1.7 | *Nature*.

[9] Ultrapotent antibodies against diverse and highly transmissible SARS-CoV-2 variants (science.org).

[10] mRNA vaccine-elicited antibodies to SARS-CoV-2 and circulating variants | *Nature*.

[11] Convalescent-Phase Sera and Vaccine-Elicited Antibodies Largely Maintain Neutralizing Titer against Global SARS-CoV-2 Variant Spikes | *mBio* (asm.org).

[12] SARS-CoV-2 variants resist antibody neutralization and broaden host ACE2 usage | *bioRxiv*.

[13] The monoclonal antibody combination REGEN-COV protects against SARS-CoV-2 mutational escape in preclinical and human studies | *ScienceDirect*.

[14] Reduced neutralization of SARS-CoV-2 B.1.617 by vaccine and convalescent serum | *ScienceDirect*.

[15] Multispecific DARPin® therapeutics demonstrate very high potency against SARS-CoV-2 variants in vitro | *bioRxiv*.

[16] SARS-CoV-2 Viral Mutations: Impact on COVID-19 Tests | *FDA*.

the virologic, epidemiologic, and clinical characteristics of the Omicron variant is rapidly emerging. CDC and other federal agencies are working closely with international public health agencies to monitor the situation closely. CDC will provide updates as more information and data become available.

Public Health Response to the Omicron Variant

On December 1, 2021, the first case attributed to the Omicron variant was identified in the United States in a person who recently return from travel to South Africa. A second case was reported on December 2, 2021 in a person with no international travel history who also attended a convention in the days preceding symptom onset. Additional possible Omicron cases are under investigation. CDC's national genomic surveillance efforts are statistically powered to detect a variant that is circulating at 0.1% with 99% confidence and can monitor changes over time. CDC and the SIG are implementing several activities in response to the Omicron variant that are summarized below:

- *Implementation of Enhanced Surveillance under the National SARS-CoV-2 Strain Surveillance (NS3) Program* – In partnership with U.S. public health laboratories and the Association of Public Health Laboratories, CDC is implementing enhanced surveillance for specimens with S-gene target failures (SGTFs) by requesting public health laboratories to send SGTF specimens to CDC as quickly as possible to speed the confirmation of possible Omicron cases and subsequent virological characterization. If public health laboratories detect Omicron through state-level surveillance activities, CDC is also requesting public health laboratories send sequence-confirmed Omicron specimens to CDC for virological characterization.
  - CDC and other federal agencies continue to work with international partners to learn more about variants circulating globally and will continue to monitor all data sources closely to identify cases of Omicron in the United States.
- *Airport Surveillance Post-Arrival Testing and Sequencing* – CDC is collaborating with two commercial partners on a SARS-CoV-2 surveillance program that involves voluntary testing of arriving

international travelers at select U.S. airports. Arriving air travelers are offered[ii] pooled testing conducted in the airport and offered at-home kits for saliva sampling that are taken 3-5 days after arrival and returned to the laboratory for RT-PCR testing. All positive samples are sequenced, enabling detection of novel SARS-CoV-2 variant among travelers entering the United States. On Sunday November 28, 2021, the program began expanding to test air travelers entering the United States from southern Africa, including passengers making connections through Europe.

- *Prioritization of laboratory studies* – The SIG has prioritized laboratory studies to evaluate the impact on available medical countermeasures, such as vaccines, therapeutics, and diagnostics. These studies include assessing the ability of vaccinee and convalescent sera to neutralize the Omicron variant, the susceptibility of the variant to treatments, and the ability of vaccine-induced immunity to protect against illness and death.
- *Support for state, local, tribal, and territorial health departments* – CDC is working closely with jurisdictions to facilitate rapid, bidirectional sharing of information. CDC staff are available to provide in-person or remote technical support for the public health response to the Omicron variant, including investigations of the epidemiologic and clinical characteristics of Omicron or other SARS-CoV-2 variant infections.
- *Travel:* On Friday, November 26, 2021, the White House issued a Presidential Proclamation suspending entry from eight countries in southern Africa for foreign nationals who were physically present in those countries during the 14 days prior to travel. CDC is working to modify the current Testing Order for travel as we learn more about the Omicron variant; a revised order would shorten the timeline for required testing for all international air passengers to one day before departure to the United States. This strengthens already robust protocols in place for international travel, including requirements for foreign nationals to be fully vaccinated. CDC continues to monitor the global epidemiology of the Omicron variant. This is a rapidly evolving situation and CDC will adjust travel recommendations and

---

ii https://www.cdc.gov/coronavirus/2019-ncov/science/science-briefs/scientific-brief-omicron-variant.html#ii.

requirements, as necessary. For the most current information about travel recommendation and requirements, see International Travel.

- CDC continues to recommend:
    - All travelers should get a COVID-19 viral test 3-5 days after arrival.
    - Travelers who are not fully vaccinated should self-quarantine for 7 days, even if their test is negative. Travelers should self-isolate if they test positive or develop COVID-19 symptoms.
    - These measures are required for foreign national who are not fully vaccinated.

- *Vaccination:* The COVID-19 vaccines approved or authorized in the United States are highly effective at preventing severe disease and death, but they are not 100% effective, and some fully vaccinated people will become infected (breakthrough infection) and experience illness. For all eligible persons, the vaccine provides the best protection against serious illness and death from COVID-19.
    - Vaccines are playing a crucial role in limiting spread of SARS-CoV-2 and minimizing severe disease. As of December 1, 2021, more than 197 million Americans are fully vaccinated and more than 233 million Americans have received at least one dose, and these numbers are increasing. Low vaccination coverage may drive increases in cases, which also increases the chances that variants could emerge.
    - Everyone 5 years and older is eligible for COVID-19 vaccination.
    - If you have received the first dose of a two dose primary vaccine series, you should get your second dose as close to the recommended 3-week or 4-week interval as possible.
    - Everyone ages 18 years and older should get a booster shot when they are eligible.
    - Data from clinical trials showed that a booster shot increased the immune response in trial participants who finished a Pfizer-BioNTech or Moderna primary series 6 months earlier or who received a J&J/Janssen single-dose vaccine 2 months earlier. With an increased immune response, people should have improved protection against COVID-19, including variants such as the Delta variant, which currently represents greater than 99% of circulating viruses in the United States. For Pfizer-BioNTech

and J&J/Janssen, clinical trials also showed that a booster shot helped prevent COVID-19 with symptoms.

- *Mitigation:* Given what we know, layered prevention strategies are needed to reduce the burden of Delta, Omicron, and all other SARS-CoV-2 variants. As we continue to build the level of vaccination nationwide and globally, we must also use all the prevention strategies available, including masking, improving ventilation, distancing, handwashing, and testing to slow SARS-COV-2 transmission and stop the COVID-19 pandemic. CDC recommends that everyone ages 2 years or older, including those who are fully vaccinated, wear masks in public indoor places where the COVID-19 Community Level is high.

Chapter 9

COVID-19 Omicron Variant: What You Need to Know*

Centers for Disease Control and Prevention

Omicron in the United States

CDC is working with state and local public health officials to monitor the spread of Omicron. As of December 20, 2021, Omicron had been detected in every U.S. state and territory and continues to be the dominant variant in the United States.

What We Know about Omicron

CDC has been collaborating with global public health and industry partners to learn about Omicron, as we continue to monitor its course. We are continuing to evaluate how easily it spreads, the severity of illness it causes, and how well available vaccines and medications work against it.

Spread

The Omicron variant, like other variants, is comprised of a number of lineages and sublineages. The three most common lineages of Omicron currently are BA.1, BA.1.1 and BA.2.

* This is an edited, reformatted and augmented version of CDC- Centers for Disease Control and Prevention Publication, updated March 29, 2022.

In: A Closer Look at the COVID-19 Variants
Editor: Richard D. Hylton
ISBN: 979-8-88697-170-5

The Omicron variant spreads more easily than earlier variants of the virus that cause COVID-19, including the Delta variant. CDC expects that anyone with Omicron infection, regardless of vaccination status or whether or not they have symptoms, can spread the virus to others.

Symptoms

Persons infected with the Omicron variant can present with symptoms similar to previous variants. The presence and severity of symptoms can be affected by COVID-19 vaccination status, the presence of other health conditions, age, and history of prior infection.

Severe Illness

Omicron infection generally causes less severe disease than infection with prior variants. Preliminary data suggest that Omicron may cause more mild disease, although some people may still have severe disease, need hospitalization, and could die from the infection with this variant. Even if only a small percentage of people with Omicron infection need hospitalization, a large volume of cases in a community could overwhelm the healthcare system which is why it's important to take steps to protect yourself.

Vaccines

COVID-19 vaccines remain the best public health measure to protect people from COVID-19 and reduce the likelihood of new variants emerging. This includes primary series, booster shots, and additional doses for those who need them.

Current vaccines protect against severe illness, hospitalizations, and deaths due to infection with the Omicron variant. However, breakthrough infections in people who are vaccinated can occur. People who are up to date with their COVID-19 vaccines and get COVID-19 are less likely to develop serious illness than those who are unvaccinated and get COVID-19.

Treatments

Scientists are working to determine how well existing treatments for COVID-19 work. Some monoclonal antibody treatments are less effective against Omicron's BA.2 lineage, but continue to work against BA.1 and BA.1.1 lineages. Other non- monoclonal antibody treatments remain effective against Omicron. Public health agencies work with healthcare providers to ensure that effective treatments are used appropriately to treat patients.

We Have the Tools to Fight Omicron

Vaccines

Getting vaccinated and staying up to date with COVID-19 vaccines is the best way to protect yourself and others against the Omicron variant.

CDC recommends that everyone 5 years and older protect themselves from COVID-19 by getting vaccinated. Everyone ages 12 years and older should stay up to date on their COVID-19 vaccines and get a booster shot when eligible.

Masks

Well-fitting masks offer protection against all variants.

- In general, people do not need to wear masks when outdoors.
- If you are sick and need to be around others, or are caring for someone who has COVID-19, wear a mask.
- If the COVID-19 Community Level where you live is:
  - Low
    - Wear a mask based on your personal preference, informed by your personal level of risk.
  - Medium
    - If you are at risk for severe illness, talk to your healthcare provider about wearing masks indoors in public.
    - If you live with or will gather with someone at risk for severe illness, wear a mask when indoors with them.

    - If you are 2 or older, wear a well-fitting mask indoors in public, regardless of vaccination status or individual risk (including in K-12 schools and other community settings).
- High
    - If you are at risk for severe illness, wear a mask or respirator that provides you with greater protection.

Testing

- Two types of tests are used to test for current infection: nucleic acid amplification tests (NAATs) and antigen tests. NAAT and antigen tests can tell you if you have a current infection.
- Self-tests can be used at home or anywhere, are easy to use, and produce rapid results.
    - If your self-test has a positive result, isolate and talk to your healthcare provider.
    - If you have any questions about your self-test result, call your healthcare provider or public health department.
- Individuals can use CDC's COVID-19 Viral Testing Tool to help determine what kind of test to seek.
- Your test result will only tell you if you do or do not have COVID-19. It will not tell you which variant caused your infection. Visit your state, tribal, local, or territorial health department's website for the latest local information on testing.

It is important to use all tools available to protect yourself and others.

What CDC is Doing to Learn about Omicron

Virus Characteristics

CDC scientists are working with partners to study data and virus samples that may answer important questions about the Omicron variant. CDC will provide updates as new information becomes available.

Variant Surveillance

In the United States, CDC uses viral genomic surveillance to track COVID-19 variants, to more quickly identify and act upon these findings to best protect the public's health. CDC established multiple ways to connect and share viral genomic sequence data being produced by CDC, public health laboratories, and commercial diagnostic laboratories within publicly accessible databases maintained by the National Center for Biotechnology Information (NCBI) and the Global Initiative on Sharing Avian Influenza Data (GISAID). Findings from CDC's variant surveillance are updated on CDC's COVID Data Tracker.

Science Brief

Omicron Lineage Variant(s) (i.e., Pango lineages B.1.1.529, BA.1, BA.1.1, BA.2, BA.3):

On November 24, 2021, South Africa reported the identification of a new COVID-19 variant, B.1.1.529, to the World Health Organization (WHO). B.1.1.529 was first detected in specimens collected on November 11, 2021 in Botswana and on November 14, 2021 in South Africa.

Emergence of Omicron

CDC has been using viral genomic surveillance throughout the course of the pandemic to track COVID-19 variants, and inform public health practice.

- November 24, 2021: A new variant of COVID-19, B.1.1.529, was reported to the World Health Organization (WHO). This new variant was first detected in specimens collected on November 11, 2021 in Botswana and on November 14, 2021 in South Africa.
- November 26, 2021: WHO named the B.1.1.529 Omicron and classified it as a Variant of Concern (VOC).
- November 30, 2021: The United States designated Omicron as a Variant of Concern.
- December 1, 2021: The first confirmed U.S. case of Omicron was identified.
- December 21, 2021: BA.2 was first identified in the United States from a sample collected on December 14, 2021, in New Jersey.

Index

S

T

U

V

W